HD
7256
.U5
M 87
1996

D1239091

A Career and Life Planning Guide for Women Survivors:

Making the Connections Workbook

A Career and Life Planning Guide for Women Survivors:

Making the Connections Workbook

Patricia A. Murphy, Ph.D.

S$_L^t$

St. Lucie Press
Delray Beach, Florida

Copyright © 1996 St. Lucie Press, Inc.
ISBN: 1-57444-021-7
Library of Congress Catalog Card Number: 94-073030

Lectures and Training Seminars
   Patricia A. Murphy offers lectures for survivors and training seminars for counselors and attorneys. Please contact Dr. Murphy at (505) 466-3694 or FAX at (505) 466-0349.

All rights reserved. No part of this publication may be reproduced, stored in a retrieval system or transmitted in any form or by any means, electronic, mechanical, photocopying, recording or otherwise, without the prior written permission of the publisher.

Printed and bound in the U.S.A.

All rights reserved. Authorization to photocopy items for internal or personal use, or the personal or internal use of specific clients, is granted by St. Lucie Press, Provided that $.50 per page photocopied is paid directly to Copyright Clearance Center, 222 Rosewood Drive, Danvers, MA, 01923 USA. The fee code for users of the Transactional Reporting Service is ISBN: 1-57444-021-7 1/96/$100/$.50. The fee is subject to change without notice. For organizations that have been granted a photocopy license by the CCC, a separate system of payment has been arranged.

   The copyright owner's consent does not extend to copying for general distribution, for promotion, for creating new works, or for resale. Specific permission must be obtained from St. Lucie Press for such copying.

PERMISSION TO REPRINT the "Diagnostic Criteria for 309.81 Post-traumatic Stress Disorder," from the *Diagnostic and Statistical Manual of Mental Disorders, Fourth Edition*, Washington, DC, 1994, was granted by the American Psychiatric Association. "Complex Post-traumatic Stress Disorders," the material quoted from *Trauma and Recovery*, 1992, by Judith Lewis Herman, M.D. was granted by Basic Books, A Division of Harper Collins Publishers, Inc. Permission to quote from *The Dinner Party: A Symbol of Our Heritage*, 1979, Anchor Books, *Embroidering Our Heritage: The Dinner Party Needlework*, 1980, Anchor Books, and *Through the Flower: My Struggle As A Woman Artist*, 1977, Anchor Books, was granted by Judy Chicago. Colleen Gibbins graciously allowed an excerpt from her letter of June 6, 1993 to the author to be quoted.

Direct all inquiries to:
   St. Lucie Press, Inc.
   100 E. Linton Blvd., Suite 403B
   Delray Beach, Florida, 33483.
   Phone: (407) 274-9906
   Fax: (407) 274-9927

S$_L^t$

St. Lucie Press
Delray Beach, Florida

about the cover

The image of the Empress Theodora (ca. 508-546, Byzantium) who ruled equally with her husband, the Emperor Justinian, is from a ceramic plate on Judy Chicago's, *The Dinner Party*. Theodora helped raise the status of women in marriage, improved the divorce laws in their favor, passed laws protecting women from mistreatment by their husbands, and established shelters for women used in prostitution.

The Dinner Party, a symbolic history of the achievements of women in Western Civilization is scheduled to be exhibited at the UCLA/Armand Hammer Museum in the Spring of 1996. The exhibition will examine the impact of this monumental tribute to women's achievements since its premier exhibition in San Francisco in 1979.

© Judy Chicago, *The Dinner Party*, 1979, Black and white version of full color photograph by Donald Woodman.

dedication

This book is for women with disabilities acquired by traumatic abuse, and for women whose pre-existing disabilities have been compounded by the experience of traumatic abuse.

May they use Title I of the Americans With Disabilities Act of 1990 to transform the workplace so that they may take their rightful place in the worlds of money, work, and power.

every woman is the re-weaver of her own life
by
Patricia A. Murphy

There is a knot inside which we find EVERY WOMAN.
And Every woman must become a weaver and a re-weaver of her own life,
Or else she will be bound tighter and tighter.

In her struggles she may sever a thread or lose one,
But she must have them all to weave her life into
An integrated whole, a pattern of her own.

Every woman is the re-weaver of her own life.

And the knot is the tangle of work, money, sexuality, and being.
When we say *women and money,* we are stuck with *gold digger, whore,*
And *women have all the money anyway.*
When we say *women and sexuality,* we follow the tangle back to
women and work,
And *women and money,*
Or to the *World's Oldest Profession.*

When we say *women and being,* we find that we don't say *women and being.*
Women's being is not recognized. Women as workers are not recognized.
Women's need for and producers of money is not recognized.
Women's sexuality as separate from men, money, and work is not recognized.

The method by which women's non-being is enforced and maintained is through the
abuse of women as children and as adults.
By rape on the job, by rape in marriage, by rape on a date, by rape on the street,
By battering in childhood, by battering in marriage. By sexual assault in marriage,
By sexual assault in childhood.
By murder in private and public places.

We are in the midst of a great revolution.
By the year 2000 women will be one half of the waged labor market.
Women are now *beings-in-the world* as never before.
The assault on women's being is escalating.

Every woman is the re-weaver of her own life.
This book is for Every woman.

table of contents

confidentiality

The work in this workbook is drawn from the stories women have told me in my years of practice as a vocational expert and vocational rehabilitation counselor. The stories are true. Most stories are composites of many stories. Every effort has been made to protect the privacy of women who may have interacted with me over the years. Anyone finding themselves in this workbook should not be alarmed. It's just that your story is not unique. The traumatic abuse of women and girls in our society is epidemic.

acknowledgments

My thanks go to Jeanne Simonoff, my long time writing friend, who put me up in her house for the Third Annual Winter Solstice Writer's Workshop so I could finish this book. To my talented copy editor, Colleen Davids Flippo. To Karen Stone who gave me the courage to think I could write about abuse and disability holistically.

about the author

Dr. Patricia A. Murphy is the author of *Making the Connections: Women, Work & Abuse*. She was awarded the John D. and Catherine T. MacAurthur Foundation's first Women's Health Policy Fellowship for Spring, 1994 at the University of Illinois Center for Research on Women in Gender in Chicago. During that time, she directed The Trauma Narratives and Americans with Disabilities Act Writing Project. This participatory action research project resulted in the monograph, *The Edge of A Large Hole: Writings on the Request for Reasonable Accommodation under the Americans with Disabilities Act of 1990*. She is the founder and director of The Making the Connections Project, as an affiliate of the Union Institute Center for Women, Washington, DC The Project's purpose was to bring the vocational rehabilitation analysis to the anti-abuse communities and traumatic abuse analysis to the rehabilitation communities. In July 1994, at the Reframing Women's Health Summer Institute sponsored by the University of Illinois at Chicago Center for Research on Women and Gender, The Making the Connections Project was transformed into the Making the Connections Intercultural Network, an international advocacy organization addressing the issues of women, work, disability, abuse, and violence. Dr. Murphy is the winner of the 1991 Most Innovative Rehabilitation Procedure Award given to her by the National Association of Rehabilitation Professionals in the Private Sector.

section I: the tools – gathering the words of power

When women accept the responsibility for evaluating and continually reevaluating their assumptions about knowledge, the attention and respect that they might once have awarded to the expert is transformed. They appreciate expertise but back away from designating anyone an expert without qualifying themselves. An evaluation of experts is not only possible but is an important responsibility that they assume. For most constructivists, true experts must reveal an appreciation for complexity and a sense of humility about their knowledge.

Belenky, Clinchy, Goldberger, & Tarule, 1986, p. 139

one

introduction

This book can be used successfully by itself. It is also intended to be the companion book to *Making the Connections: Women, Work & Abuse,* (Murphy, 1993) which laid the groundwork for analyzing how abuse can create disability and/or vocational impairment. *Making the Connections: Women, Work & Abuse* also pointed out that the profession of vocational rehabilitation counseling had already evolved a methodology and an analysis for serving survivors of trauma, but that until now, this analysis and practice was designed to meet the needs of male survivors of combat or of industrial accidents.

If *Making the Connections: Women, Work & Abuse* can be considered as a description of the problem, then *A Career and Life Planning Guide for Women Survivors: Making the Connections Workbook* is the solution. Or, to put it another way, the vocational rehabilitation plan. The purpose of this book is to assist women survivors of abuse in creating and directing their own vocational plans whether or not these efforts take place in state departments of rehabilitation; workers' compensations systems; long-term disability systems; the dissolution of marriage process; domestic tort, sexual harassment, civil sexual assault, and civil incest lawsuits; work and welfare programs such as the JOBS program arising out of the Family Services Act; or as part of an individually determined recovery process.

When I described my plan for the writing of these books to Laura Davis, the nationally recognized author of *The Courage to Heal Workbook*, she asked me why I did not include men. She writes, "I've come to learn that most of the (abuse) issues faced by male and female survivors are the same" (Davis, 1990). I agree with this assessment. However, what is not the same for women and men in our society is work, and the differences are profound. They include inequities in education and employment, wages and income, pensions and Social Security benefits. The invisible and unwaged work of women is still not shared by men in any significant way, and includes housework, child care, and elder care. Women employed in the waged labor market contribute an average of 22 hours per week to household services as contrasted to the 11 hours per week contributed by men (Field, 1989). Women's discontinuous work patterns in the waged labor market mean that women spend almost a decade less than men in the waged labor markets, and the life expectancies of men and women differ by approximately eight years (U.S. Department of Labor Bureau of Labor Statistics, February, 1986). In short, men work in the waged labor market longer, and die sooner than women. This means retirement planning for women and men also differs. The result is that "almost 15% of all women aged 65 and over live below the poverty level, a figure twice that of elderly men. ... contributing to older women's poverty are discriminatory Social Security practices, the lack of pension coverage and personal savings, and the pressure for early retirement" (Rayman & Allshouse, December, 1990).

This book is meant to be used as *part* of the recovery process from abuse. Recovery may involve individual counseling, group therapy, 12-Step programs including AA, NA, AL-ANON, ACA, massage, physical therapy, and other body work techniques, medical interventions, journal work, volunteer and paid staff work in rape crisis centers, and domestic violence shelters systems. Recovery from the abuse experience(s) can be as complex as recovery from any traumatic accident or catastrophe such as an earthquake, automobile accident, or prisoner of war experience. Injuries may be both physical and psychological. They may be onetime events as in a rape experience, or multiple occurrences as in childhood sexual abuse or sexual harassment on the job, taking place over a period of months or years. Some survivors may have multiple abuse experiences which are both onetime events and repeated incidents of abuse (e.g., a rape survivor who experiences domestic violence over a period of months or years, or a rape survivor who has been used in prostitution for an extended period of time).

Whatever your experience of abuse has been, the workbook is designed to assist you with understanding how this abuse may have created vocational impairment in your life and how to set about correcting or compensating for that impairment. Therefore, this workbook is for survivors of all ages whose abuse experience(s) may have taken place 50 years or a few months ago.

Rehabilitation counselors, vocational experts, psychotherapists, rape crisis counselors, caseworkers, employment counselors, and shelter workers may also find the workbook a useful tool in the provision of services to abuse survivors.

prostitution and wife battering as forms of slavery

Since this workbook is also for women and girls who are recovering from the experience of being used in prostitution, the question of prostitution as work arises. Prostitution is defined in this book as violence against women and girls, not work. I consider prostitution as a form of slavery. I do not see it as a career choice. The use of the word *slavery* in this context is important since it allows us to address both the issue of violence against women and girls and the fact that prostitution is thought of as *work* by some people (even feminist thinkers). The definition of female sexual slavery used in this book was written by Kathleen Barry (1979):

> *Female sexual slavery is present in all situations where women or girls cannot change the immediate conditions of their existence; where, regardless of how they got into those conditions they cannot get out; and where they are subject to sexual violence and exploitation.*

Joyce E. McConnell's (1992) brilliant and provocative essay, *Beyond Metaphor: Battered Women, Involuntary Servitude and the Thirteenth Amendment,* also explores the concept of female slavery even though she is writing about married women subjected to battering and marital rape by their husbands. It is interesting to note that "when Congress debated the Thirteenth Amendment and its prohibitions against slavery and involuntary servitude, anxious members inquired whether it would alter the traditional relationship of husband and wife." (McConnell, 1992) A similar attitude was revealed by Congress when the word *sex* was added to the Civil Rights Bill of 1964 by southern senators who expected that adding gender to the Bill would lead to its defeat. It did not, and the Civil Rights Bill of 1964 has been important in women's struggle for equal rights. McConnell's work challenges the courts to extend the protection of the Thirteenth Amendment to battered women.

In fact, it appears to be impossible to separate discussions of prostitution, marriage, and slavery from each other. In *International Feminism: Networking Against Female Sexual Slavery: Report of the Global Feminist Workshop to Organize Against Traffic in Women* (Barry, 1984, p. 34-35) we find, "marriage and dependency is central to both the devaluation and marginalization of woman's labor and the exploitation of women in prostitution." And McConnell (1992) in a review of current cases demonstrating involuntary servitude echoes Barry's definition of female sexual slavery. She writes "the cases demonstrate two well-settled principles of involuntary servitude: a relationship freely entered into can convert to one of involuntary servitude, and where the level of coercion meets a legal standard, the mere fact that one held in involuntary servitude does not avail herself or himself of an opportunity to escape does not defeat a finding that the person is held in involuntary servitude."

The connections among the American enslavement of millions of Africans, the involuntary servitude of the battered woman, and global female sexual slavery in systems of prostitution are too complex and too numerous to be addressed here. Although recent scholarship, as exemplified by Robert William Fogel (1989) in *Without Consent or Contract: The Rise and Fall of American Slavery*, offers vitally important information and analyses leading to a more sophisticated understanding of the systems of female slavery, it is important to remember that the Thirteenth Amendment of 1865 did not even address the rights of enslaved African and African-American women. We women (African-American, European-American, Asian-American, Hispanic-American, Native American) have only had the vote since 1920. The idea of equal opportunity in employment and education was considered to be a joke in 1964, and in 1994 we still don't have an Equal Rights Amendment.

some thoughts on the word *disability*

Disabled women, no matter the subject being explored, are an invisible population.

Rebecca Grothaus, 1985, pp. 124-130

My use of the word *disability* in the discussion of abuse dynamics is not meant to obscure or obliterate the vulnerability of women and girls with disabilities to childhood and adult battering and sexual assault. Instead, I would like to suggest that the Disabled Women's Movement has much to teach women survivors of abuse, and the anti-abuse movements have much to offer the Disabled Women's Movement.

The notion that abuse may create disabling physical and psychological conditions which may or may not lead to vocational impairment is a new (even if obvious) concept. What is new about this concept is that a vocational impairment analysis applies to women as well as to combat veterans and male industrially injured workers. It may feel uncomfortable or stigmatizing to label oneself as *disabled*. It may feel like one more insult piled on top of years of verbal-emotional abuse. However, to avoid this term is possibly to deprive yourself of services, benefits, and damage awards which may be your due. Women with disabling conditions who have also experienced abuse may face a similar dismay at identifying themselves as rape or incest survivors, or battered women. The same principles apply—you may not be able to use services and benefits available to abuse survivors without identifying yourself within these groups.

In 1990, the United States Congress passed the Americans With Disabilities Act (ADA). The Civil Rights Act of 1964 and the Rehabilitation Act of 1973 formed the legislative base for the ADA. The Civil Rights Act of 1964 allowed for the filing of sexual and racial discrimination suits in order to correct inequities in employment and education. The ADA extends these rights to *Qualified Disabled Individuals*. The ADA is not an affirmative action statute. Instead, it seeks to dispel stereotypes and assumptions about disabilities, and to ensure equality of opportunity, full participation, independent living and economic self-sufficiency for disabled people. The law prohibits covered entities from excluding people from jobs, services, activities or benefits based on disability, and the ADA provides penalties for discrimination.

Women who have sustained physical and/or psychological injuries as a result of rape, battering, incest, sexual exploitation in prostitution or in cults, and sexual harassment in the workplace may be determined as *Qualified Disabled Individuals* under the ADA. Similarly, women with disabling conditions prior to their abuse experience(s) may find that although they have been able to function in the labor market, or in educational programs with their disability, they will need to assert the rights gained under the ADA after being abused.

In either case, the filing of a law suit (domestic tort, civil incest, civil sexual assault, sexual harassment, or ADA suits) will necessitate addressing in written and verbal testimony the damage and injury you have suffered. The terms *disability* and *disabling condition* may be used by vocational experts, attorneys, juries, judges, and other experts. These terms may refer to both physical and psychological injuries.

All rehabilitation delivery systems (e.g., workers' compensation, state departments of rehabilitation, long-term disability insurance, Social Security Disability Insurance) use an eligibility determination process which is based on definitions of disability. It has been historically easier to obtain services and benefits for physical disabilities than for psychological disabilities, and until 1980, abuse survivors were frequently diagnosed inappropriately. The inclusion of post-traumatic stress disorder in the *American Psychiatric Diagnostic and Statistical Manual* (1980) meant that survivors finally had a sensible diagnosis which could be used by the various rehabilitation and legal systems. Judith Lewis Herman (1992) has proposed an additional diagnosis for the 4th revision of this important manual, *complex post-traumatic stress disorder*. This diagnosis applies to survivors who have experienced abuse over a period of months or years. Both post-traumatic stress disorder (PTSD) and complex post-traumatic stress disorder (CPTSD) will be used extensively in this workbook as part of *an empowerment process for survivors.* We've come a long way. We now have language which describes the experience(s) of abuse and the resulting trauma. This language allows survivors to be determined as *disabled* or eligible for damage awards in law suits or in rehabilitation benefit systems. Abuse survivors have a right to use all of these systems.

definitions of work

The word *work* in this Workbook always refers to both waged and unwaged work, even though I attempt to identity both types of work whenever possible. Waged work refers to the exchange of labor for wages. Unwaged work refers to the work of child care, elder care, housework, gardening, driving, shopping, and all the other tasks which women do in their "spare time" when they are not working for wages (such as they are) in the labor market. Therefore, when I use the term *vocational impairment* I refer to the damage caused by traumatic abuse to both the waged and unwaged work lives of women.

RESOURCE – Marilyn Waring. (1988). *If Women Counted: A New Feminist Economics.* New York: Harper & Row.

how to use this workbook

This book is designed to help you explore your identity as a worker, and more importantly, as a woman worker. There are three parts to the Workbook. The first part is *The Tools – Gathering the Words of Power.* Therefore, the second chapter in this section is a *Glossary of Terms* because if you should chose to manipulate (or find yourself in the midst of) complex and esoteric rehabilitation and/or legal systems as part of your recovery process, having access to the language and terminology of bureaucratic systems is the first step in empowering yourself in these systems. The third chapter in this section is *Naming the Trauma.* The purpose of this chapter is to develop a common vocabulary of the traumatic experience with the professionals who may be helping you in your recovery process. The fourth chapter, *Reclaiming My Innocent Body*, is structured to assist you in increasing your resistance to the pervasive denial of the vulnerability of the body . The fourth chapter, *Overcoming Verbal- Emotional Abuse,* is designed to assist you in claiming the power of definition, naming, and affirmation as your birthright.

The second part of the Workbook is *The Process – Moving Through the Flower.* This section has four chapters, including an introduction to the work of the artist Judy Chicago. The *Making Your Work Visible* chapter is a way of looking at your achievement history within a context of women's history. *Analyzing, Respecting, & Celebrating Your Work* is a method of empowering yourself by using the official language of the *Dictionary of Occupational Titles* and by celebrating your treasure trove of skills. *Understanding Your Vocational Impairment* is a challenging chapter which allows you to take a giant step forward in your growth by starting from where you stand now. All of the exercises in this section are based on the concepts of Judy Chicago as documented in her books, and in her massive collaborative art projects, most notably, *The Dinner Party Project. The Dinner Party* is a symbolic history of women in Western Civilization interpreted through 39 place settings, each honoring a woman or goddess. These are executed in ceramic, china-painting and needlework and are set on an open table. The table rests on a lustered, white porcelain floor, upon which are inscribed the names of 999 women who made a mark on history. The floor, like the table, is configured as an equilateral triangle, an ancient symbol of the Goddess and the feminine (Through the Flower, undated). The purpose of this section is to enable you to claim your heritage as a working woman in Western Civilization.

The third part of the Workbook is *The Plan – Re-Weaving Your Own Life and Work*. This section also has four chapters, including an introduction. They are, *Making the Frame* which empowers you to spin a yarn, a web to hold your dreams. *Stretching the Self* describes that process of carefully, with great patience and love, making a life for yourself, and *Weaving A Life* suggests that you have the power of the goddess within you to confront the most pernicious of bureaucratic systems. The purpose of this section is to empower you to become the artist, the weaver, the architect of your own life.

TIPS

TIPS are found throughout the workbook. They are designed to be safety first reminders.

RESOURCES

Resources are located in the workbook where and when you need them. For example, in the *Glossary of Terms* under the term *Civil Incest Case* you will find:

RESOURCE – *Legal Resource Kit: Incest and Child Sexual Abuse,* NOW Legal Defense and Education Fund, 99 Hudson Street, New York, NY 10013-2815, (212) 925-6635 FAX (212) 226-1066.

TIP

Go to *The Affirmation Exercises for Overcoming Verbal-Emotional Abuse* if you start feeling overwhelmed by the *Glossary of Terms,* or when you are feeling overwhelmed by any of the material in this book.

TIP

Remember, using the *Glossary of Terms* over and over while you read this book or are trying to deal with a bureaucratic system is sign of intelligence. This is because the first rule of recovery is always safety first. Feeling overwhelmed is not safe. It is okay to read this book any way you please, in small doses, from the back, in sections, out loud in a group, or to one other person, or out loud to yourself, with your therapist or rehabilitation counselor or vocational expert. If reading is difficult for you, have someone else read it to you.

TIP

The 1994 *The Courage to Heal, Third Edition* by Ellen Bass and Laura Davis has a 52-page Resource Guide with its own table of contents. Rather than reinventing the very fine wheel developed by Bass and Davis, I refer you to their 1994 Resource Guide. This Guide is suitable for women who have been abused as adults as well as children. The Guide includes books, magazines, organizations, films, newsletters, and topic headings of interest to survivors.

two

glossary of terms

Each of us is here now because in one way or another we share a commitment to language and to the power of language, and to the reclaiming of that language which has been made to work against us.

Audre Lorde, 1984

Ableism: A belief that being able-bodied or mentally capable or emotionally well makes one superior to a person with disabilities. A prejudice.

ADA: See *Americans with Disabilities Act.*

Age earning cycle: As we age, our earnings decline. One way to defeat the age earning cycle is through education. Statistically the more education we have, the more opportunities we have to flatten the age earning cycle or to keep our earnings higher longer. This is true for women and men.

Americans with Disabilities Act (ADA): The Americans with Disabilities Act (ADA) of 1990 extends federal civil rights protection in employment, public services and transportation, public accommodations, telecommunications, and miscellaneous provisions to people who are considered disabled. It is built upon the Rehabilitation Act of 1973 and the Civil Rights Act of 1964. The purpose of the ADA is to provide "a clear and comprehensive national mandate for the elimination of discrimination against individuals with disabilities."

RESOURCE – The ADA Compliance Guide (1990) is an important resource for those who wish to keep up to date on the rapid evolution of ADA case law. The monthly newsletter is well-written. Thompson Publishing Group, 1725 K Street NW, Suite 200, Washington, DC 20006, 1 (800) 424-2959.

Aptitude test: A standardized test designed to predict an individual's ability to learn certain skills (e.g., The Wide Range Achievement Test [WRAT]).

Award: See *Damage Award.*

Battered child syndrome: Dr. Henry Kempe organized an multidisciplinary conference in 1961, *Battered Child Syndrome*. His efforts paved the way for the medical profession's recognition of the physical abuse of children. Neglect including dehydration, malnourishment, and anemia are the most common signs of child battering, followed by multiple fractures, and cerebrospinal injury. Battered children are withdrawn, terrified, and fail to express emotion.

RESOURCE – Karp, L., & Karp, C. L. (1989). *Domestic Torts: Family Violence, Conflict and Sexual Abuse.* Colorado Springs, CO: Shepard's/McGraw-Hill, Inc.

Battered Woman Syndrome (BWS): The BWS is defined by Douglas (1987) as "the (1) traumatic effect of victimization by violence; (2) learned helplessness deficits resulting from the interaction between repeated victimization by violence and the battered woman's and others' reactions to it, and (3) self-destructive coping responses to the violence." A subcategory of post-traumatic stress disorder (PTSD).

Civil incest case: A civil suit brought by one person against another person or persons for monetary damages based on damages caused by incest.

RESOURCE – Crnich, J. E., & Crnich, K. A. (1992). *Shifting the Burden of Truth: Suing Child Sexual Abusers–A Legal Guide for Survivors and Their Supporters.* Lake Oswego, Oregon: Recollex Publishing.

RESOURCE – Legal Resource Kit: Incest and Child Sexual Abuse, NOW Legal Defense and Education Fund, 99 Hudson Street, New York, NY 10013-2815, (212) 925-6635 FAX (212) 226-1066.

Civil Rights Act of 1964: Rights that guarantee to all citizens equal opportunities (in employment, schooling, housing, or voting) regardless of race, religion, sex, or national origin.

Civil sexual assault case: A civil suit brought by one person against another person or persons (hotel, apartment, or building owner) for monetary damages based on damages caused by rape/sexual assault.

RESOURCE – National Coalition Against Sexual Assault, (NCASA), P.O. Box 21378, Washington, DC 20009, 202/483-7165.

Civil suit: Private rights and remedies sought by action or suit distinct from criminal proceedings. See *Civil Incest Case, Civil Sexual Assault Case, Domestic Tort.*

Complex Post-traumatic Stress Disorder: Complex post-traumatic stress disorder (CPTSD) is under consideration for inclusion in the fourth edition of the diagnostic manual of the American Psychiatric Association. It is based on seven diagnostic criteria, and was named and developed by Judith Lewis Herman in her book *Trauma and Recovery* (1992). See *Post-traumatic Stress Disorder.* The major difference between these disorders appears to be that complex post-traumatic stress disorder involves the experience of trauma which took place over an extended period of time as opposed to a one-time experience (e.g., a rape).

Consumer mental health movement: A civil rights movement of persons using mental health systems.

Co-researcher: Instead of referring to someone interviewed for the purposes of research as a *subject,* the phenomenological or qualitative researcher acknowledges the interviewee as a fellow explorer, as a *co-researcher.* That is, in *Making the Connections: Women, Work & Abuse,* I did not assume that I was the only one with the expertise on the subject of women, work, and abuse. Every survivor who reads and completes all or part of the workbook is also a co-researcher.

Covered entity: The Americans with Disabilities Act Title I applies to all employers except those with fewer than fifteen employees (fewer than 25 until July 26, 1994). Covered entities include employers (private and public sector), employment agencies, labor organizations, and joint labor-management committees.

Creative process: Used in the career and life planning process to mean the ability to approach problem solving not just as an intellectual task but as a creative experience which engages the heart, mind, body, and soul.

Damage award: A monetary award based on damages. Damages can include money for past and future medical expenses, past and future psychotherapy/counseling expenses. Compensation for past lost wages, future lost wages, expenses related to a vocational plan including tuition, books, supplies, uniforms. Compensation for the loss of pleasure in life or hedonic damage award. See *Hedonic Damage Award.*

RESOURCE – Scalise, J. J. (Ed.).(1989, Fall). *The Professional Reader: Estimating Future Lost Earnings As a Consequence of Injury.* Volume 1, Number 3, Athens, GA: Elliot & Fitzpatrick, Inc.

Delayed memory debate: This debate was created by the False Memory Syndrome Foundation, and has been given credibility by the mass media. The debate positions therapists providing therapy to child abuse survivors with post-traumatic stress disorder and complex post-traumatic stress disorder symptoms versus those who insist that therapists "brainwash" survivors into recovering memories of child abuse.

RESOURCE – The daughter (Dr. Jennifer J. Freyd) of Pamela Freyd, founder of the False Memory Syndrome Foundation, has written a paper, *Theoretical and Personal Perspectives on the Delayed Memory Debate,* which refutes the claims of the False Memory Foundation. The paper can be obtained from The Making The Connections Project at 86 Monte Alto Road, Santa Fe, NM 87505. The cost of this Project Working Paper is $5.00.

Disabled Women's Movement: A civil rights movement of women with physical and mental disabilities arising out of the Consumer Mental Health and the Independent Living Movements, and energized by the passage of the Americans with Disabilities Act of 1990. Women with disabilities have found that neither the Women's Movement nor the Disability Civil Rights Movement have included them in their agendas in any significant way. See *Consumer Mental Health Movement, Independent Living Movement.*

RESOURCE – Health Resource Center for Women with Disabilities, Rehabilitation Institute of Chicago, 345 East Superior, Chicago, IL 60611, (312) 908-7997. Administrative Director, Judy Panko Reis. *Strengthening the Links – Stopping the Violence* (1994) by Leanne Cusitar of the DisAbled Women's Network (DAWN) Toronto, 180 Dundas Street West, Suite 120, Toronto, Ontario, M5G 1Z8. DAWN is probably the world leader in examining the consequences of that fact that women with disabilities are 150% more likely to have someone sexually assault them than non-disabled women!

Disability: See *Introduction, Some Thoughts on the Word Disability.* The definition of disability referred to in this book is taken from the Americans with Disabilities Act (ADA) and is defined as a physical or mental impairment that substantially limits one or more of major life activities of a person; a record of such an impairment; or being regarded as having such an impairment. See *Physical Impairment, Mental Impairment, Major Life Activities, Record of Impairment, Regard As Impaired, Substance Abuse.*

Domestic tort: A civil suit brought by one spouse against another for damages caused by assault and battery, marital rape, emotional injury, defamation.

RESOURCE – Karp, L. & Karp, C. L. (1989). *Domestic Torts: Family Violence, Conflict and Sexual Abuse.* Colorado Springs, CO: Shepard's/McGraw-Hill, Inc.

Earning capacity: Refers to the ability to make money in the waged labor market based on a past history of earnings and/or a statistical estimate drawn from government tables which are based on gender, race, and age.

Employment law: Refers to a body of law which includes the Americans with Disabilities Act, Civil Rights Act of 1964 (Title VII - Race and Sex Discrimination), Civil Rights Act of 1991, Sex Harassment Law, Age Discrimination in Employment Act, and state laws which address these issues. Excludes workers' compensation law.

Essential functions: See *Americans with Disabilities Act, Disability, Nonessential Functions, Qualified Disabled Individual, Reasonable Accommodation.* The definition of essential functions on a job will be determined on a case by case basis as lawsuits are filed under the ADA. Some elements in determining essential functions include the existence of a job category just to perform that function; the number of workers available to perform the function; the function requires specialized skills such as flying a plane or interpreting a foreign language; the employer's judgment as to which functions are essential.

Exertional limitation: A restriction which affects the capability to perform an exertional activity such as sitting, standing, walking, pushing, pulling, lifting and/or carrying. (Social Security Administration, Office of Hearings and Appeals, 1990, February).

False Memory Syndrome/False Memory Syndrome Foundation: See *Delayed Memory Debate*. There is no diagnosis in the recognized listing of mental disorders (*The Diagnostic & Statistical Manual of Mental Disorders* published by the American Psychiatric Association) as *false memory syndrome.* The term is an invention of the False Memory Syndrome Foundation.

RESOURCE – The 1994 *The Courage to heal, Third Edition–Revised and Updated* by Ellen Bass and Laura Davis, This edition is particularly important since the authors have written a 57-page response to the False Memory Syndrome Foundation and their supporters titled, "Honoring the Truth: A Response to the Backlash." Laura Bass and Ellen Davis have suffered the chilling attempt to censor their First Amendment rights as writers because of frivolous lawsuits filed against them by backlash support.

Family Services Act of 1988: An overhaul of the AFDC system tying work to welfare, and requiring mothers to participate in work and/or training programs when the youngest child reaches the age of two years, or risk losing welfare support.

Female sexual slavery: See *Introduction, Prostitution and Wife Battering As Forms of Slavery* "Female sexual slavery is present in *all* situations where women or girls cannot change the immediate conditions of their existence; where, regardless of how they got into those conditions they cannot get out; and where they are subject to sexual violence and exploitation" (Barry, 1979).

Feminist vocational rehabilitation model: A feminist or womanist vocational rehabilitation model is women-centered. That is, based on the lives of women and on the reality of pervasive violence which permeates so many women's lives, distorting every woman's efforts to develop, possess, and nurture a work identity in waged and unwaged work. This model also acknowledges that abuse leads to physical and psychological injury which can be disabling. For a complete description of this model see *Making the Connections: Women, Work, and Abuse*, pp. 207-214 (Murphy, 1993).

Heavy work: This is work involving the lifting of no more than 100 pounds at a time with frequent lifting or carrying of objects weighing up to 50 pounds. A worker who can perform *heavy work,* can also perform *medium, light,* and *sedentary work* (Social Security Administration, Office of Hearings and Appeals 1990, February).

Hedonic damage award: An award based on the loss of pleasure in life and/or pain and suffering. Life has a value above and beyond lost wages or lost professions. The use of vocational experts in offering testimony as to the hedonic value of a loss of a work identity or the loss of profession or occupation because of abuse has not yet been attempted although a 1990 study provides a basis for hedonic awards for the loss of occupations (Magrowski, 1990).

RESOURCE – Magrowski, J. F. (1991). *Introduction to hedonics.* Hedonology Institute, P.O. Box 260007, St. Louis, MO 63126, (314) 394-8563.

Independent living movement: A civil rights movement by persons with severe (usually) physical disabilities who demand the right to full and independent lives in a barrier-free, accessible society.

Interest inventory: A inventory of likes and dislikes which allows for systematic vocational exploration (e.g., The Strong Campbell Interest Inventory).

Interspousal immunity: "The common law rule that prohibited one spouse from suing the other for personal injuries has been seriously eroded or abrogated in most jurisdictions over the past 20 to 30 years." (Karp & Karp, 1989, 1993, June) See *Domestic Tort.*

Job market: See *Labor market.*

Labor force: "The labor force consists of the employed and unemployed but not the underemployed, the marginally employed, the would-be-employed, and certainly not those who work in the informal sector or who work as housewives" (Waring, 1988. pp. 25-27).

Labor market: Also known as the *job market* where one sells one's labor for wages and benefits.

Labor market survey: A survey of available jobs in a given geographical area by reviewing classified advertising in a local newspaper, by telephoning employers listed in the yellow pages in the local telephone book, by using government resources located in your local library or community college, and by examining other listing of job openings such as job boards at a college or at local employment office.

RESOURCE – *The Economic Consequences of Child Sexual Abuse in Women,* an unpublished dissertation by Batya Hyman of April, 1993, is available from The National Clearinghouse on Child Abuse and Neglect, P.O. Box 1182, Washington, DC 20013-1182 for around $25. This dissertation is a well-documented piece of quantitative research which reveals that childhood sexual abuse can mean loss of earning capacity as adults in the waged labor markets. *The Effects of Violence on Work and Family*, a research project directed by doctoral candidate, Susan Lloyd, with the Center for Urban Affairs and Policy Research at Northwestern University, 2040 Sheridan Road, Evanston, IL 60208-4100, will be completed in June, 1995. A telephone survey of 1000 randomly selected adult women in the West Humboldt Park area of Chicago is "expected to add significantly to what is known about women's employment, about the impact of male and street violence on individual women, work, and family life, and about the effects of violence on individual behavior and community well-being."

Light work: This is work involving lifting no more than 20 pounds at a time with frequent lifting or carrying of objects weighing up to 10 pounds. A job is classified as *light work* when it requires a significant amount of walking or standing – the primary difference between *sedentary* and *light work*. A job is also in this category when it involves sitting most of the time with some pushing and pulling of arm-hand or leg-foot controls. (e.g. mattress sewing machine operator) (Social Security Administration, Office of Hearings and Appeals, 1990, February).

Major life activities: The definition is based on the Americans with Disabilities Act (ADA) as follows: self-care, manual tasks, walking, seeing, hearing, speaking, breathing, learning, working. In *Making the Connections: Women, Work & Abuse,* I documented how abuse can impair or completely destroy the ability to work or learn. One co-researcher in my study had lost the sight in her left eye as a result of battering. This precluded her from participating in her occupation of nursing because of her lack of depth perception.

Malingering: The pretense that one is ill or disabled in order to avoid physical work, or work in general. The most widely used psychological test in the world, *The Minnesota Multiphasic Inventory (MMPI)*, has a scale which purports to measure malingering. This issue frequently arises in disability determinations (Social Security, workers' compensation) where no "objective" evidence of disability can be documented in medical reports.

Marital rape: "Under the common law, rape was defined as the unlawful carnal knowledge of a woman, *not a spouse,* forcibly and against her will. According to the common law rule, there is irrevocable implied consent by married women to sexual intercourse with their husbands. A husband, therefore, could never be found guilty, in a criminal trial, of raping his wife. By 1987, however, approximately 60 percent of the states had removed their marital exemption from their criminal rape statutes" (Karp and Karp, 1989). In other words, in some states it is still legal for husbands to rape their wives.

Medium work: This is work involving lifting of no more than 50 pounds at a time with frequent lifting of objects weighing up to 25 pounds. Sitting may occur intermittently (Office of Hearings and Appeals, Social Security Administration, 1990, February).

Mental impairment: The definition is based on the Americans with Disabilities Act (ADA) as follows: mental or psychological disorder including emotional or mental illness, specific learning disabilities, mental retardation, organic brain syndrome. Post-traumatic stress disorder (PTSD) and complex post-traumatic stress disorder (CPTSD) have been found to be common outcomes of the trauma of rape, battering, and incest. See *post-traumatic stress disorder, complex post-traumatic stress disorder, battered woman syndrome, and rape trauma syndrome.*

RESOURCE – Herman, J. L. (1992) *Trauma and Recovery.* New York: Basic Books.

Negative worker traits: Traits which may constitute vocational impairment resulting in the inability to sustain or obtain employment in the waged labor market. Some post-traumatic stress disorder and complex post-traumatic stress disorder symptoms may be negative worker traits. Negative worker traits may also render education and skilled work abilities unusable in waged and unwaged work.. See *Worker Traits* for an explanation of the difference between skills and traits.

Nonessential functions: See *Americans with Disabilities Act, Disability, Essential Functions, Qualified Disabled Individual.* These functions will also be defined on a case by case basis as lawsuits are brought under the ADA, but include marginal tasks in a job such as driving for a telemarketing salesperson.

Nonexertional impairment: An impairment which does not directly affect the ability to sit, stand, walk, lift, carry, push or pull. Includes impairments which affect the mind, vision, hearing, speech, and the use of the body to balance, stoop, kneel, crouch, crawl, reach, handle, and use of the fingers for fine activities (Social Security Administration, Office of Hearings and Appeals 1990, February).

Physical capacity: See *Residual Functional Capacity.*

Physical demands: The physical demands of jobs are classified in *The Dictionary of Occupational Titles* as **sedentary work, light work, medium work, heavy work,** and **very heavy work** (See each category of work for more detail.) (Social Security Administration, Office of Hearings and Appeals, 1990, February).

Physical impairment: The definition is based on the Americans with Disabilities Act (ADA) as follows: physiological disorder, contagious disease, cosmetic disfigurement, or anatomical loss in one or more system. Systems include neurological, musculoskeletal, respiratory, cardiovascular, reproductive, digestive, gentiourinary, hemic, lymphatic, skin, endocrine. Common injuries resulting in physical impairment for domestic violence survivors include musculoskeletal injuries such as injuries to the spine in the neck, middle and lower back. The prevalence of traumatic brain injuries experienced by domestic violence survivors is still unknown. However, at every *Making the Connections Meetings and Seminars* series I have presented, rehabilitationists specializing in traumatic brain injury have been present.

This would indicate that head injury resulting from battering is not unusual. Incest survivors may experience digestive disorders. Rape survivors may have genito-urinary damage as the result of vaginal tears. Sexually transmitted diseases which may impair many or all physical systems are possible outcomes of the rape trauma.

RESOURCE –Subscription to *Journal of Interpersonal Violence*, PO Box 5084, Newbury Park, CA 91359.

Physical work capacity: One's capacity for meeting the physical demands of waged and unwaged work. See *Residual Functional Capacity*. See *Physical Demands*.

Post-traumatic stress disorder: Post-traumatic stress disorder (PTSD) is defined in the American Psychiatric Association's fourth edition of its diagnostic manual (DSM-IV). Its numerical code is 309.81. See the chapter titled, *Naming the Trauma*. See *complex post-traumatic stress disorder*. The major difference between these disorders appears to be that PTSD is a one-time traumatic event as opposed to an extended period of traumatic experience(s) (e.g., months or years of wife battering).

Prostitution: See *female sexual slavery*.

RESOURCE – The Council for Prostitution Alternatives (CPA), 65 SW Yamhill, 2nd Floor, Portland, OR 97204, (503) 223-4670, takes the position "that prostitution is not a profession... It is abusive, dehumanizing, and often life threatening."

Qualified individual with a disability (QID): See *Americans with Disabilities Act, Disability, Essential Job Functions, Reasonable Accommodation*. The Americans with Disabilities Act (ADA) offers protection to those who have a disability as defined by the ADA, under Title I of the ADA, who also qualify to perform the essential functions of a job, with or without a reasonable accommodation by the employer.

Rape Trauma Syndrome (RTS): A subcategory of Post-traumatic Stress Disorder (PTSD). May involve a "compounded reaction to rape trauma" (Burgess and Holstrom, 1979) and "Unresolved sexual trauma" (Burgess and Holstrom, 1985).

Reasonable accommodation: See *Americans with Disabilities Act, Undue Hardship*. This is a very broad-based definition which covers equal opportunity in the job application process; accommodations which enable qualified disabled individuals to perform essential job functions including making facilities accessible and usable, restructuring jobs, allowing part-time or modified work schedules, acquiring or modifying equipment or devices, providing readers or interpreters, and reassigning an employee to a vacant position. Employers do not have to provide reasonable accommodation if they face undue hardship. Qualified individuals with disabilities must request the reasonable accommodation from the employer.

RESOURCE – *The Edge of a Large Hole: Writings on the Request for Reasonable Accommodations Under the Americans with Disabilities Act of 1990* by Patricia A. Murphy. Center for Research on Women and Gender, UIC, 1640 W. Roosevelt Road, Room 207 (M/C 980), Chicago, IL 60608. (312) 413-1924.

Record of impairment: This definition is taken from the Americans with Disabilities Act (ADA) and notes that the individual has a history of impairment or a record of having been misclassified as having an impairment. This might be an important consideration for an abuse survivor who has been inappropriately diagnosed as *manic-depressive, borderline personality,* or *schizophrenic.* Survivors with a history of substance abuse may also face difficulties. Labeling may create discrimination in the workplace. If so, the Americans with Disabilities Act provides the right to sue based on that discrimination.

Regard as impaired: The definition is taken from the Americans with Disabilities Act (ADA) and notes that the individual has an impairment not limiting a major life activity, but is treated as disabled by the covered entity, or no impairment, but treated as disabled by the covered entity. See *Record of Impairment.* For example, abuse survivors who have experienced cosmetic disfigurement which does not create an impairment in the ability to work may face discrimination in locating work because of the disfigurement. Under the ADA, such a person would meet the definition for disability.

Rehabilitation Act of 1973: This Act served to implement an earlier disability-related law, the Architectural Barrier Act of 1968, which requires federal and federally assisted facilities to be accessible to and usable by the physically disabled. In 1977, Section 504 of the Act required federal grantees to make their programs and jobs accessible to disabled people. The Act is the precursor of the ADA, and the ADA borrows much of its terminology from this Act.

Rehabilitative alimony: Alimony usually awarded to spouses in long-term marriages who have been out of the waged work world for extended periods of time. Also known as *spousal support* in some states. The purpose of the alimony is to assist the supported spouse while she (or he) gets training so that she is able to become self-sufficient. This type of alimony is time-limited. Having a detailed vocational plan when requesting rehabilitative alimony is a good strategy. Otherwise, a judge will decide what you should have, and he will base this on his ideas and not your needs.

Relationship or association with a disabled person: See *Americans with Disabilities Act.* This provision of the ADA prohibits employers from discriminating against a non-disabled employee or applicant because of any association or relationship that person might have with a disabled individual. Whether or not battered women will be able to use this provision of the ADA when employers do not either retain an employee or hire an applicant who is associated with a battering husband or partner will only be discovered in a court of law. For example, a recent study of men identified as perpetrators of domestic violence indicated that 61 percent had a history of head injury (Allison, M., 1993, March/April).

Residual functional capacity: The maximum degree to which a worker retains the capacity for sustained performance of the physical and mental requirements of jobs (Social Security Administration, Office of Hearings and Appeals, 1990, February).

Sedentary work: This is work involving the lifting of no more than 10 pounds at a time and occasionally lifting or carrying articles like docket files, ledgers, and small tools. Although sedentary jobs involve sitting, they also require a certain amount of standing and walking to carry out job duties (Social Security Administration, Office of Hearings and Appeals, 1990, February).

Semi-skilled work: See *Skill Levels.*

Skilled work: See *Skill Levels.*

Skill levels: This is a work classification whereby work is defined as unskilled, semi-skilled, or skilled according to the skill requirements of the occupation. *Unskilled work* requires little or no judgment to perform simple duties that a can be learned on the job in a short period of time. *Semi-skilled work* requires some skills but does not require performing the more complex work duties. *Skilled work* requires the performance of complex work duties (Social Security Administration, Office of Hearings and Appeals, 1990, February).

Slavery: See *Female Sexual Slavery.*

Spousal support: See *Rehabilitative Alimony.* Each state has its own precise legal definitions of these terms. State department of rehabilitation (DR) or state department of vocational rehabilitation (DVR) Every state in the United States has an agency whose mission is to serve the disabled in education and employment. The ADA has, for the first time, mandated that these agencies assist disabled individuals who wish to advance in their employment.

Statute of limitations: A legal rule which states how long a civil suit can be filed after an injurious act has taken place. This is of particular importance to survivors of child battering and child sexual assault. Each state has its own rules (e.g., in California civil actions for recovery of damages from child sexual abuse are now limited to eight years after the child reaches the age of 21, or three years from the date the survivor discovers that the psychological injury or illness was caused by the abuse.) See *Delayed Memory Debate* and *False Memory Syndrome.*

Stockholm Syndrome: The Traumatic Bond "The Stockholm Syndrome was first identified in 1973, after four people held captive in a Stockholm bank vault for six days became attached to the robbers. The hostages actually came to perceive the police as the *bad guys* and the captors as the *good guys*. "This bonding may be a universal response to inescapable violence. Battered women are no more worthy of blame than a hostage kidnapped off the street" (Karp & Karp, 1993, June).

Substance abuse: The Americans with Disability Act does not include the current, illegal abuser of drugs and alcohol as a disabled person. However, persons recovered from substance abuse may be covered under the ADA. Substance abuse is also considered a common complication of post-traumatic stress disorder and complex post-traumatic stress disorder.

Transferability of skills: Skills demonstrated by past waged and unwaged work performance which can meet the skill demands of other semi-skilled and skilled jobs in which the same or lesser degree of skill is required (Social Security Administration, Office of Hearings and Appeals, 1990, February).

Undue hardship: See *Americans with Disabilities Act, Qualified Individual with a Disability, Reasonable Accommodation.* This is another broadly based term which will be clarified as lawsuits are filed under the ADA. Employers are not obligated to provide reasonable accommodation in the workplace if the accommodation creates an undue hardship for the employer which would involve significant difficulty (such as changing the entire nature of the business) or expense (such as requiring a small employer to perhaps purchase costly equipment).

Unskilled work: See Skill levels.

Unwaged work: This term was created by the feminist economist Marilyn Waring to refer to the unpaid work of child care, elder care, nursing care, housework, gardening, and all the invisible work in our society which is unpaid. Waring asserts that this unpaid, unwaged labor deserves to be called *work* (Waring, 1988).

Very heavy work: This is work involving the frequent lifting of objects weighing 50 pounds or more. A worker who can perform *very heavy work*, can also perform *heavy, medium, light,* and *sedentary work* (Social Security Administration, Office of Hearings and Appeals, 1990, February).

Violence Against Women Act of 1993: Attached to the hotly-debated, highly political Crime Bill, the Violence Against Women Act "was more than six years in the making.... It is the most comprehensive piece of federal legislation the government has enacted to combat the growing problem of violence against women. The act authorizes $1.6 billion to protect women from abusers, punish batterers and improve the way the criminal justice system handles domestic violence and other forms of violence against women (Tripp, 1994, November)." The resurgence of a Republic House and Senate may not bode well for the actual disbursement of the $1.6 billion authorized by Congress just a few months before the elections.

Vocational expert: An expert used in legal settings to provide testimony and consultation to the attorneys, juries, judges. Legal settings include divorce or dissolution of marriage cases regarding rehabilitative alimony issues; personal injury cases for lost earning capacity issues; civil sexual assault, sexual harassment, civil incest, and domestic tort cases for lost earning capacity and hedonic or noneconomic award damages; and ADA cases for vocational impairment and disability issues leading to lost earnings and other noneconomic damages..

Vocational impairment: Damage to one's ability to perform in the waged and unwaged worlds of work. Disability does not necessarily mean that an individual is vocationally impaired or excluded from all work (e.g., a person with paraplegia who uses a wheelchair can perform many jobs as well as function capably in the unwaged work of child care and housework). However, such jobs as auto mechanic or professional ice skater may be impossible for a person with this disability.

Vocational plan or vocational rehabilitation plan: A detailed, usually written, plan describing on-the-job training, supported employment, formal training in a business school, trade school, or college. Formal plans written in workers' compensation systems, state departments of rehabilitation, long-term disability health insurance coverage usually include supporting documentation of the individual's ability to benefit from the training (vocational testing, physical capacities evaluation) and documentation regarding the practicality of the plan (labor market surveys). The costs of the plan are also carefully noted.

Vocational rehabilitation: A process which involves overcoming physical and/or mental disabilities in order to return to work in a usual and customary occupation, a modification of the usual and customary occupation, an alternative job with the same employer, a change in occupation, or the obtaining of waged work for the first time. See *A Feminist Vocational Rehabilitation Model.*

Waged work: Labor which is exchanged for wages (Waring, 1988, pp. 25-27).

Woman: This word refers to all women in our complex, diverse culture, and is not meant to refer to dominant-culture European-American women only.

Womanist: This is a term preferred by African-American women who identify the term *feminist* as referring to dominant-culture European-American white women.

Women's Health Movement: Also know as the Reframing Women's Health Movement. This is a broadly based multidisciplinary movement to reframe women's health in the education and practice of physicians and other health care professionals. Although the Women's Health Movement emerged with the rise of feminism in the late 60s, the resurgence of this movement in the 90s was partially brought about by the notorious Physicians Health Study sponsored by the National Institute of Health which conducted research leading to a finding that aspirin may have a prophylactic effect on cardiovascular disease in men. Since the leading cause of death among women in the United States is cardiovascular disease, basing a research sample on 22,071 men and 0 women seems, in the mildest terms, highly inappropriate. The Women's Health Movement also recognizes violence against women as a major health problem for women.

Work: See *Unwaged Work* and *Waged Work.* My definition of work includes all productive activity whether it takes place in the labor market or in the home.

Worker: A primary identity in American culture. Women are workers. This identity is earned in both waged and unwaged work.

Workers' compensation: A legal/medical/rehabilitative process by which workers injured on the job are compensated for their injuries. Each state has its own body of workers' compensation law. There is also federal workers' compensation for federal employees.

Worker traits: Traits are not the same as skills. See *Skill Levels*. See *Transferability of Skills.* Skills refer to experience and demonstrated proficiency with particular tasks or jobs. Worker traits, to be relevant, must have been used in connection with a work activity. Thus the trait of alertness is connected with the work activities of close attention to watching machine processes, inspecting, testing, tending or guarding; and the traits of coordination and dexterity with the use of hand or feet for the rapid performance of repetitive work tasks. Skills exist in occupations found in the arts and sciences, and in crafts or trades. A musician requires both a good sense of pitch and fine finger dexterity (traits) to play a piece of music by ear without error (skill); a lab researcher may require acute vision (trait) to identify a particular bacteria found in a culture (skill); a machinist must rely on perception of size and shape (trait) to cut material within certain tolerances (skill) (Social Security Administration, Office of Hearings and Appeals, 1990, February).

My Additions to the Glossary of Terms

TIP

As bureaucracy changes (and it always does) new terms and buzz words emerge. You may wish to keep track of these terms as you move through the mazes of bureaucratic rehabilitative/medical/ legal systems.

_____

_____

_____

_____

_____

_____

_____

_____

_____

_____

_____

_____

_____

_____

_____

_____

_____

_____

_____

_____

_____

_____

_____

_____

_____

_____

_____

_____

_____

_____

_____

_____

three

_____

naming the trauma

Where language and naming are power, silence is oppression, is violence.

Adrienne Rich, 1977

The listing of post-traumatic stress disorder (PTSD) in the *Diagnostic and Statistical Manual (DSM-III-R)* in 1980 meant that the damaging effects of trauma were *finally* officially acknowledged by the American Psychiatric Association. Since 1980, there has been an explosion of books, articles, and research on trauma. However, some researchers have suggested that although PTSD is a useful description for survivors of one traumatic event, it is not so useful a description for survivors of prolonged, repeated trauma. Judith Lewis Herman (1992) developed a new diagnosis for the 4th revision of the *DSM (DSM-IV)*. Her proposed description would not replace the post-traumatic stress disorder diagnosis (PTSD), but would take its place as an added diagnosis called complex post-traumatic stress disorder (CPTSD).

When I wrote *Making the Connections: Women, Work & Abuse,* Dr. Herman's complex post-traumatic stress disorder diagnosis or description was not available. Therefore, I could not refer to it in that book even though my co-researchers and I had discovered that an abuse history of one isolated traumatic event was the exception rather than the rule. When I reviewed Dr. Herman's CPTSD diagnosis, I immediately saw that it was a more accurate description of the traumatic abuse experience for most survivors than the PTSD diagnosis. When I prepared the vocational impairment commentary to be added to the diagnostic criteria for each trauma description, I was struck by the richness and depth of the CPTSD description. This meant a correspondingly rich and deep description of the vocational impairment impact which results from traumatic abuse.

Therefore, we will examine both PTSD and CPTSD in this chapter since this Workbook is for the use of survivors of both onetime traumatic experiences, such as a onetime rape, and multiple and/or prolonged experiences of trauma, such as wife battering or the incest trauma.

a cautionary note on working with vocational rehabilitation counselors

Vocational rehabilitation counselors have a unique relationship to disabling conditions. Even though it is part of their job to understand and be aware of a wide range of disabling conditions, which can be both physical and psychological, they are not the professionals who diagnose or treat the disabling condition. Rehabilitation counselors generally work with other professionals such as medical doctors, psychologists, psychiatrists, physical therapists, and occupational therapists. The job of the vocational rehabilitation counselor is to understand how a disabling condition impairs an individual's work life and how that impairment can be overcome.

In fact, your rehabilitation counselor may deliberately choose a counseling strategy which suppresses dialogue between the two of you about your disability. This is because counselors are frequently confronted with clients who may have already spent months or even years in endless recitations of pain, medical interventions, and the catastrophes which result from disabling conditions such as loss of job, marriage, and money. This is no bad reflection on clients who may be forced into such recitations in order to receive benefits in the various medical-legal systems such as workers' compensation or state departments of rehabilitation. In any of these systems, the job of the rehabilitation counselor is to assist the client in focusing on ability, not disability or what is sometime referred to as *residual functional capacity.* This just refers to the ability remaining to an individual after sustaining an injury or disability. The best rehabilitation counselors focus on ability and how that ability will engender a new work life for the client.

Such a counseling strategy is not appropriate for trauma survivors. The opposite strategy needs to take place, focusing on the nature of the injury until both parties share a common knowledge base. Then the process of switching focus from disability to ability can occur.

The injurious effects of trauma are still unknown to most people, including rehabilitation counselors and abuse survivors. This is partly due to the fact that the post-traumatic stress disorder diagnosis has only been officially available since 1980, and partly due to the deeply ingrained belief by many people that survivors of trauma of any sort are suspect. General George S. Patton gained infamy when he struck a shell-shocked or traumatized combat soldier during World War II; Patricia Bowman's testimony in the William Kennedy Smith rape trial was not considered credible and Smith was acquitted; the Senate Judiciary Committee's handling of Anita Hill's

> **TIP**
>
> If the idea of *Naming Your Trauma* is overwhelming, refer to the chapter, *Overcoming Verbal-Emotional Abuse.* You may wish to create an affirmation to use before doing the work in this section. A suggested affirmation is *I (your name) am safe now.* I also suggest doing the *Naming the Trauma Exercises* with your recovery group, your rehabilitation counselor, or with your therapist.

sexual harassment allegations against the Supreme Court nominee Clarence Thomas was a study in the discounting of the sexual harassment experience; Francine Hughes ended up burning her husband to death in his bed because no one would take the danger to herself and her children from the brutal violence of Mickey Hughes seriously; a great deal of the current literature on child witness testimony still centers on Freud's notorious conclusion that most incest survivors are lying, or fantasizing. In short, we are still struggling against the deeply ingrained idea that trauma survivors are lying, fantasizing, or exaggerating their symptoms or injuries.

This means that a shared vocabulary between you and your counselor regarding the nature of trauma is vital for a productive relationship. The PTSD listing in the *DSM-IV* and Herman's (1992) CPTSD give us that vocabulary, a language we can all share. It is useful for counselor and client to sit down together and go over the trauma symptoms, keeping in mind the particular situations which may work against your rehabilitation process. For example, a colleague of mine used this technique with a woman who had been diagnosed with PTSD as a result of being held up at gunpoint more than once in her work as a grocery checker. The claims examiner in the workers' compensation case was quite impatient with the trauma survivor when she mentioned that she was uneasy with going to a school a few blocks away from the store where she had been held up. This lack of ease had also been triggered by the sexist comments of male students at the school when she had come onto the premises for an entrance examination. The survivor had a hard time explaining herself, and dithered back and forth with her rehabilitation counselor about the level of her discomfort. Once the counselor and the survivor sat down together and went over the PTSD symptoms as listed in the *DSM-IV* diagnostic

> **TIP**
>
> It is highly unlikely that a rehabilitation counselor in a workers' compensation system or a state department of rehabilitation office will be able to provide you with psychotherapeutic counseling services regarding your trauma. Your rehabilitation counselor will expect to work with you and your therapist while you are in rehabilitation.

criteria, the survivor was able to acknowledge her deeply rooted fear of going to that particular school. The counselor then sent a copy of the PTSD diagnostic criteria to the claims examiner along with her report, and a more appropriate rehabilitation training program was found. The resistance by the claims examiner evaporated in the face of concrete knowledge of trauma and its resulting vocational impairment. The counselor and the survivor have moved on beyond detailed discussions of trauma, but they can now refer back to that conversation as part of the rehabilitation process, and this allows them both to focus on the vocational goal with the least amount of stress.

Therefore, one of the purposes of this chapter is to give you, the trauma survivor, the language to use with your rehabilitation counselor. Sharing this chapter with your rehabilitation counselor may be a useful strategy in developing a productive relationship. Explain to your counselor that you wish to share a common language with her/him so that you may get on with your vocational rehabilitation in the most positive, creative manner possible.

RESOURCE – If you sense that your counselor is still having trouble taking you seriously, ask the counselor to order the *PTSD Interview (PTSD-1): DSM-III-R Version.* This instrument was developed by Charles G. Watson, Ph.D. of the Veteran's Administration. It can be administered by rehabilitation counselors to screen for a possible post-traumatic stress disorder diagnosis. (Such a diagnosis would have to be confirmed by a clinical psychologist or psychiatrist to be used as an official determination of disability.) Order from The Making The Connections Intercultural Network, 86 Monte Alto Road, Santa Fe, NM 87505 at a cost of $5.00.

TIP

If you are feeling intimidated by your counselor even though you think she/he is okay, repeat an affirmation before each meeting with your counselor. A suggested affirmation is, *I (your name) am a competent person in charge of my own life.* The counselor is there to help you, not to run your life. Another useful affirmation might be, *My counselor (her/his name) wants to help me, (your name).* These affirmations address the negative belief system that you don't deserve help, or that no one, not even your counselor is to be trusted.

TIP

If your counselor persists in not developing a shared vocabulary regarding trauma, ask for a new counselor.

The second, and perhaps more important purpose for this chapter is for you to name your own trauma so that you have the best understanding of your trauma experience possible. This trauma inventory may also assist you in creating affirmations because the PTSD and CPTSD diagnostic criteria can also be seen as descriptions of negative thoughts and experiences common to trauma survivors. The chapter, *Overcoming Verbal-Emotional Abuse,* is designed to assist you to identify negative beliefs you hold about yourself, transform them into affirmations, and then use the affirmations in the process of healing repetition.

At this time, the Battered Woman Syndrome, the Rape Trauma Syndrome, the Stockholm Syndrome, the Battered Child Syndrome, and the Child Abuse Accommodation Syndrome are all considered to be subcategories of PTSD. I have chosen to not use these subcategories in the Workbook for two reasons. First, even though Dr. Herman's (1992) CPTSD was not adopted into the DSM-IV, it gives us a method of including some of the subleties and complexities of the subcategories without having to grapple with five or six descriptions of trauma instead of two, as represented by the post-traumatic stress disorder and the complex post-traumatic stress disorder descriptions.

Secondly, if you should choose to participate in (or find yourself in the middle of) any rehabilitation system, it is more useful to use the recognized trauma language adopted by the psychiatric profession. This language will be the most effective in obtaining an official determination of disability which would then make you eligible for whatever services and benefits are available under Social Security Disability, workers' compensation systems, state departments of rehabilitation, or long-term disability insurance policies. The PTSD language also promotes the idea that rape survivors, combat survivors, concentration camp survivors, earthquake victims, and child battering victims may have similar responses to their respective traumas. In other words, your trauma experience is not just a "woman" thing.

TIP

Refer to the *Glossary of Terms* for definitions of the PTSD subcategories such as Battered Woman Syndrome, Rape Trauma Syndrome, Stockholm Syndrome.

Naming the Trauma Exercises

Post-traumatic STRESS DISORDER
(The post-traumatic stress disorder diagnostic criteria 309.81 is quoted from the *DSM-IV*, published by The American Psychiatric Association in 1994.)

A.

The person has been exposed to a traumatic event in which both of the following were present:

1. The person experienced, witnessed, or was confronted with an event or events that involved actual or threatened death or serious injury, or a threat to the physical integrity of self or others.

2. The person's response involved intense fear, helplessness, or horror. Note: In children, this may be expressed instead by disorganized or agitated behavior.

My experience of trauma is:

_____

_____

_____

_____

Instruction: You may have experienced only some or all of the symptoms listed below. If you have not had the experience described, simply go on to the next symptom on the list.

B.

The traumatic event is persistently re-experienced in at least one of the following ways:

1. Recurrent and intrusive distressing recollections of the event (in young children, repetitive play in which themes or aspects of the trauma are expressed).
Yes_____**No**_____.

I also experience(d): _____

_____

_____

_____

_____

Possible Vocational Impairment: Difficulty in learning in school, on the job, or new tasks. Underemployment or not working up to vocational capacity. Disruption in early education leading to interrupted or delayed completion of education.

Because of these recollections, I experience(d) the following damage to my education, my work life:

_____

_____

_____

2. Recurrent distressing dreams of the event. Note: In children, there may be frightening dreams without recognizable content. **Yes**_____ **No**_____.

I also experience(d): _____

_____

_____

_____

Possible Vocational Impairment: Lack of rest which impairs mental clarity on the job or at school or in my work as a parent.

Because of these distressing dreams, I experience(d) the following damage to my education, my work life (waged and unwaged):

_____

_____

_____

3. Sudden acting or feeling as if the traumatic event were recurring (includes a sense of reliving the experience, illusions, hallucinations, and dissociative flash-back episodes, including those that occur upon awakening or when intoxicated). Note: In young children, trauma-specific reenactments may occur.
Yes_____ No_____.

I also experience(d): _____

_____

_____

_____

Possible Vocational Impairment: Difficulty in concentrating/focusing on school assignments and/or work and housekeeping tasks. Difficulty in socializing with others and caring for my children.

Because of these sudden actions or feelings of the trauma recurring, I experience(d) the following damage to my relationships with others at school, in my home, on the job:

_____

_____

_____

4. Intense psychological distress at exposure to internal or external cues that symbolize or resemble an aspect of the traumatic event.
Yes_____ No_____.

I also experience(d): _____

_____

_____

_____

Possible Vocational Impairment: Difficulty in being in places where the trauma took place such as an office building, or parking structure, or at parties or events such as office parties, business conferences, or other work settings.

Because of my distress, I avoid the following work or school settings, events, and/ or anniversaries:

_____

_____

_____

5. *Physiological reactivity on exposure to internal or external cues that symbolize or resemble an aspect of the traumatic event.* **Yes** _____   **No** _____

I also experience(d): _____

_____

_____

_____

Possible Vocational Impairment: Chronic illnesses leading to absenteeism on the job, at school. Possible substance abuse to control symptoms also leading to absenteeism on the job, at school.

Because I'm (sick or under the influence) much of the time, (I can't work regularly, I'm disabled, I can't get through school, I have trouble supervising my kids). I have developed the following physical symptoms because of the trauma.

_____

_____

_____

_____

C.

Persistent avoidance of stimuli associated with the trauma or numbing of general responsiveness (not present before the trauma), as indicated by at least three of the following:

1. Efforts to avoid thoughts or feelings associated with the trauma.
Yes_____ **No**_____.

I also experience(d): _____

_____

_____

_____

Possible Vocational Impairment: Suppression of the creative impulse. Difficulty in concentrating or focusing on new learning in the home, educational endeavors, and on the job. Fatigue.

Because of my efforts to avoid thoughts or feelings associated with the trauma, I find that my work life, my educational process, my work in the home are damaged in the following ways:

_____

_____

_____

2. Efforts to avoid activities or situations that arouse recollections of the trauma.
Yes_____ **No**_____.

I also experience(d): _____

_____

_____

_____

Possible Vocational Impairment: Inability to leave one's home to go to work or to school or to handle parenting tasks such as driving children to school and activities. Loss of occupations which may remind the victim of the trauma.

Because of my efforts to avoid activities or situations that remind me of the trauma, I have lost the following:

_____

_____

_____

3. Inability to recall an important aspect of the trauma. **Yes**_____ **No**_____.

I also experience(d): _____

_____

_____

_____

Possible Vocational Impairment: Suppression of the creative impulse. Survivor may have stopped painting, singing, dancing, writing. Loss of confidence. Suppression of the willingness to take the risk of new learning and challenge.

Because of my inability to recall aspects of my trauma, I find that I am unsure of myself at school, at work, with my children in the following ways:

_____

_____

_____

4. Markedly diminished interest in significant activities.
Yes _____ **No** _____.

I also experience(d): _____

_____

_____

Possible Vocational Impairment: No interest in planning for the future. Difficulty in making commitments or in completion of education, classes, projects.

Because of my lack of interest in things, the damage to my education, my work has been:

_____

_____

_____

5. Feeling of detachment or estrangement from others. **Yes** _____ **No**_____.

I also experience(d): _____

_____

_____

_____

Possible Vocational Impairment: Damage to social skills needed for interaction in educational and work settings. Damage to parenting skills.

Because of my feelings of detachment and estrangement from others, I find that my interactions with my children, my fellow students, my co-workers are damaged as follows:

_____

_____

_____

6. Restricted range of affect (e.g., unable to have loving feelings).
Yes _____ **No**_____.

I also experience(d): _____

_____

_____

_____

Possible Vocational Impairment: Damage to social skills needed for interaction in work, school, and in the family. Suppression of pleasure, joy, and creativity in the activities of school, work, and home.

Because of my lack of feelings, I find that my pleasure in work, home, and school is damaged in the following ways:

_____

_____

_____

7. Sense of a foreshortened future (e.g., does not expect to have a career, marriage, or children, or a long life). **Yes** _____ **No** _____ .

I also experience(d): _____

_____

_____

_____

Possible Vocational Impairment: Difficulty in completing education including classes and degrees. Difficulty in keeping commitments including being on time, or keeping promises. Career and life planning efforts appear useless or impossible. May hold a deep-seated belief that one is going to die soon, so why bother? The victim may not know that she holds this belief, but acts out of it anyway.

Because I don't believe in my future, I have not completed the following educational projects:

_____

_____

_____

D.

Persistent symptoms of increased arousal (not present before the trauma), as indicated by at least two of the following:

1. Difficulty falling or staying asleep. **Yes** _____ **No** _____ .

I also experience(d): _____

_____

_____

_____

Possible Vocational Impairment: Lack of rest leading to lack of mental clarity on the job, in parenting, in classes. Fatigue leading to on the job injury or other accidents.

Because I'm so tired all the time, I find that (my work, my learning, my parenting) is damaged in the following ways:

_____

_____

_____

2. Irritability or outbursts of anger. **Yes** _____ **No** _____ .

I also experience(d): _____

_____

_____

_____

Possible Vocational Impairment: Difficulty in interactions with others, particularly supervisors or subordinates. Damage to parenting skills.

Because I'm so irritable and angry, I (have struck out at my children, yelled at my boss, lost my job, got a poor performance evaluation, have no friends at school):

_____

_____

_____

3. Difficulty concentrating. **Yes** _____ **No** _____ .

I also experience(d): _____

_____

_____

_____

Possible Vocational Impairment: Difficulty learning new tasks, performing complex and/or detailed tasks. Lack of self-confidence.

Because I have difficulty concentrating, I have problems (in school, at work, at home) as follows:

_____

_____

_____

4. Hypervigilance. **Yes** _____ **No** _____.

I also experience(d): _____

_____

_____

_____

Possible Vocational Impairment: Damage to social skills. Difficulty in risk taking, either no risks taken or the risk-taking is inappropriate.

Because I'm watching out all the time, I find that it is hard to (be close to people, concentrate on something to the exclusion of all else, socialize in strange places or at parties):

_____

_____

_____

5. Exaggerated startle response. **Yes** _____ **No**_____.

I also experience(d): _____

_____

_____

_____

Possible Vocational Impairment: Damage to social interactions. Fear of others. Fatigue.

Because I'm so easily startled (People are not comfortable with me or I'm not comfortable with them, I tired easily, and I'd rather stay home). Other problems include:

_____

_____

_____

E.

Duration of the disturbance (symptoms in B, C and D) is more than one month.
Yes _____ **No**_____.

F.

The disturbance causes clinically significant distress or impairment in social, occupational, or other important areas of functioning.
Yes _____   **No** _____

These disturbances have lasted since (approximate date or dates) _____.

Today's date is: _____

TIP

Congratulations! By naming your trauma symptoms, you have taken your power over the language used by helping professionals. Feel free to take a copy of this exercise when you interact with your counselor, therapist, or attorney. You may or may not choose to give them a copy. You may wish to use this document to refer to as notes for yourself only. This may prevent being tongue-tied or silenced when interacting with the helping professionals.

TIP

Remember that the PTSD symptoms are now accepted by the American Psychiatric Association in their publication, *DSM-IV*. The CPTSD symptoms listed below have been *proposed* by Dr. Judith Lewis Herman for inclusion in the *DSM-IV* were not accepted. Therefore, the PTSD diagnosis is currently the official diagnosis to used in determining eligibility for disability program services and benefits.

You may wish to work both *Naming the Trauma* exercises, or just the *PTSD* or the *CPTSD* exercises, or portions of either. You choose.

COMPLEX POST-TRAUMATIC STRESS DISORDER

(The complex post-traumatic stress disorder diagnostic criteria is quoted from Judith Lewis Herman [1992] in *Trauma and Recovery*, p. 121)

---

1. A history of subjection to totalitarian control over a prolonged period (months to years). Examples include hostages, prisoners of war, concentration camp survivors, and survivors of some religious cults. Examples also include those subjected to totalitarian systems in sexual and domestic life, including survivors of domestic battering, childhood physical or sexual abuse, and organized sexual exploitation.

My experience of totalitarian control over a prolonged period is:

_____

_____

_____

_____

Possible Vocational Impairment: Long absences from the waged labor market, underemployment, inability to complete or continue educational and vocational preparation, criminal record (for being used in prostitution, welfare fraud), economic deprivation (homelessness, signing over all assets), lack of external support systems, loss of social skills, physical injuries (e.g., orthopedic injuries, closed head injury, dental trauma), chronic illnesses (malnutrition, pelvic diseases, substance abuse), chronic pain syndrome, chronic fatigue.

The ways this experience of totalitarian control has damaged my education, my work life, my economic life are:

_____

_____

_____

_____

2. Alterations in affect regulation, including persistent dysphoria, chronic suicidal preoccupation, self-injury, explosive or extremely inhibited anger (may alternate), compulsive or extremely inhibited sexuality (may alternate).

My experience of persistent dysphoria (unhappiness), suicidal thoughts, explosive or sometimes inhibited anger and sexuality has been/is:

_____

_____

_____

_____

_____

Possible Vocational Impairment: Damage to social skills, (e.g., difficulty with supervision and feedback in the workplace or at school) chronic health problems including substance abuse leading to absenteeism and poor performance in school and on the job, vulnerability to inducement and/or extortion into prostitution, vulnerability to sexual harassment on the job/in education.)

My inability to handle my angry impulses, my sexual impulses, my moods has damaged my work life, my education, my economic life in the following ways:

_____

_____

_____

_____

_____

_____

_____

3. Alterations in consciousness, including amnesia or hypermnesia for traumatic events, transient dissociative episodes, depersonalization/derealization, reliving experiences, either in the form of intrusive post-traumatic stress disorder symptoms or in the form of ruminative preoccupation.

My experience of either thinking all the time about my prolonged traumatic experiences or blocking it out (sometimes leaving my body or becoming another person) can be described as follows:

_____

_____

_____

_____

_____

Possible Vocational Impairment: Difficulty concentrating on tasks, new learning in the workplace and at school, delay and/or damage to developmental skills such as reading, language development, mathematics, possible lack of work identity, stunting of the creative process.

The damage to my ability to do well in school or college, or on the job can be described as follows:

_____

_____

_____

_____

_____

_____

_____

4. Alterations in self-perception, including sense of helplessness or paralysis of initiative, shame, guilt, and self-blame, sense of defilement or stigma, sense of complete difference from others (may include sense of specialness, utter aloneness, belief no person can understand, or nonhuman identity)

My experience of prolonged traumatic abuse means the way I think about myself is:

_____

_____

_____

_____

_____

Possible Vocational Impairment: Inability to develop a work identity, possible loss of one's name, inability to take risks (e.g., launch a new career, get a college degree, borrow money), inability to make friends or enter the "old girl network" in school or at work, unable to understand or appreciate mentoring (distrusts authority or people with education or professional status), holds belief of inability to learn because of verbal-emotional abuse (e.g., being called *stupid* or *crazy*), no belief in her own transferable skills and knowledge base, may be phobic about going to school or have the idea she has no *right* to learn, experiences words as weapons and not as tools, may hold belief that she is only fit to be used in prostitution, not fit to be in the company of others.)

My perceptions of myself have prevented me from fulfilling the following educational, economic, and work goals (including the unwaged work of having children):

_____

_____

_____

_____

_____

5. Alterations in perception of perpetrator, including preoccupation with relationship with perpetrator (includes preoccupation with revenge), unrealistic attribution of total power to perpetrator (caution: victim's assessment of power realities may be more realistic than clinician's), idealization or paradoxical gratitude, sense of special or supernatural relationship, acceptance of belief system or rationalizations of perpetrator.

My relationship to the perpetrator(s) can be described as follows:

_____

_____

_____

_____

_____

_____

Possible Vocational Impairment: May move with or follow perpetrator from city to city (e.g., in a marriage or in a pimp/prostitute relationship) which disrupts education and career development, escaping from perpetrator by going underground which also disrupts education and career, allow unwaged work skills (parenting/caretaking) to be degraded, (e.g., children are abused in the name of discipline or perpetrator's special needs) accepts perpetrator's evaluation of the value of education, work, and money including the idea that having a higher level of skills, knowledge, education, work, and money than the perpetrator is a betrayal of the perpetrator, accepts perpetrator's control of money and the right to communicate with others, and holds these beliefs even if the perpetrator is dead.

Because of my relationship with the perpetrator(s) I have experienced the following losses in my work life, my education, my parenting responsibilities:

_____

_____

_____

_____

_____

6. Alterations in relations with others, including isolation and withdrawal, disruption in intimate relationships, repeated search for rescuer (may alternate with isolation and withdrawal), persistent distrust, repeated failures of self-protection.

My prolonged experience of traumatic abuse has meant that my relationships with others can be described as:

_____

_____

_____

_____

_____

_____

Possible Vocational Impairment: Loss of support systems which would allow risk taking in career development, inappropriate relationships with teachers/mentors/bosses including sexual relationships and vulnerability to sexual harassment in the workplace and in the educational process, vulnerability to inducement into prostitution (average age of entry in the U.S. is between 13 and 16 years leading to further trauma and possible life-long vocational impairment), inability to utilize mentoring or networking support in career development, underemployment by working in jobs which will insure isolation (e.g., working alone as a maid when the victim is a college graduate).

The quality of my relationships with others has effected my work life and my educational endeavors in the following ways:

_____

_____

_____

_____

_____

7. Alterations in systems of meaning including loss of sustaining faith, sense of hopelessness and despair.

My experience of hopelessness has meant that I: _____

_____

_____

_____

_____

_____

Possible Vocational Impairment: No planning for the future, difficulty completing education and long range projects, no pleasure in work, lack of passion in all endeavors, suppression of the creative impulse, no sense of the value of contribution to be made to others, expectation that work will be oppressive, routine, and without joy, expectation that others in the workplace will either be oppressive or isolating, neglects parenting/caretaking duties because of no belief in the worth of life for oneself and one's children.

The sense of hopelessness I experience has meant that my waged and unwaged work life and my educational efforts could be best described as follows:

_____

_____

_____

_____

_____

_____

Congratulations again! If you have worked all or a portion of *Naming the Trauma* exercises you have gathered some of the words of power you need for your recovery. A formerly battered woman described this process to me as "comforting, in a kind of sideways way, if you know what I mean." I do, because naming is challenging, exciting, creative, and sobering, all at the same time. Welcome to the experience of power.

> **TIP**
> The pages at the end of this chapter are summaries of *Vocational Impairment Commentary on the PTSD Diagnostic Criteria* and *Vocational Impairment Commentary on the CPTSD Diagnostic Criteria.* These summaries may be used as handouts when you do not wish to share the workbook pages you have completed, and which contain your private commentary regarding your experience of trauma with others.

Abuse is both a psychological and a physical experience. The purpose of next chapter, *Reclaiming My Innocent Body,* is to continue the process of naming the trauma, and to honor the body/mind connection, the whole person. The concluding chapter in *Part I, Overcoming Verbal- Emotional Abuse*, is designed to help you to take back the power of words, of naming, of definition. This power is your birthright, your heritage.

Vocational Impairment Commentary on the PTSD Diagnostic Criteria

---

> **POST-TRAUMATIC STRESS DISORDER**
> (The post-traumatic stress disorder diagnostic criteria 309.81 is quoted from the *DSM-IV*, published by The American Psychiatric Association in 1994.)

A.

The person has been exposed to a traumatic event in which both of the following were present:

1. The person experienced, witnessed, or was confronted with an event that involved actual or threatened death or serious injury, or a threat to the physical integrity of self or others.

2. The person's response involved intense fear, helplessness, or horror. Note: In children, this may be expressed instead by disorganized or agitated behavior.

B.

The traumatic event is persistently reexperienced in at least one of the following ways:

1. Recurrent and intrusive distressing recollections of the event (in young children, repetitive play in which themes or aspects of the trauma are expressed).

Possible Vocational Impairment: Difficulty in learning in school, on the job, or new tasks. Underemployment or not working up to vocational capacity. Disruption in early education leading to interrupted or delayed completion of education.

2. Recurrent distressing dreams of the event. Note: In children, there may be frightening dreams without recognizable content.

Possible Vocational Impairment: Lack of rest which impairs mental clarity on the job or at school or in my work as a parent.

3. Sudden acting or feeling as if the traumatic event were recurring (includes a sense of reliving the experience, illusions, hallucinations, and dissociative flashback episodes, even those that occur upon awakening or when intoxicated). Note: In young children, trauma-specific reenactments may occur.

Possible Vocational Impairment: Difficulty in concentrating/focusing on school assignments and/or work and housekeeping tasks. Difficulty in socializing with others and caring for my children.

4. Intense psychological distress at exposure to events that symbolize or resemble an aspect of the traumatic event, including anniversaries of the trauma.

Possible Vocational Impairment: Difficulty in being in places where the trauma took place such as an office building, or parking structure, or at parties or events such as office parties, business conferences, or other work settings.

5. Physiological reactivity on exposure to internal or external cues that symbolize or resemble an aspect of the traumatic event.

Possible Vocational Impairment: Chronic illnesses leading to absenteeism on the job, at school. Possible substance abuse to control symptoms also leading to absenteeism on the job, at school.

C.

Persistent avoidance of stimuli associated with the trauma or numbing of general responsiveness (not present before the trauma), as indicated by three or more of the following:

1. Efforts to avoid thoughts or feelings associated with the trauma.

Possible Vocational Impairment: Suppression of the creative impulse. Difficulty in concentrating or focusing on new learning in the home, educational endeavors, and on the job. Fatigue.

2. Efforts to avoid activities or situations that arouse recollections of the trauma.

Possible Vocational Impairment: Inability to leave one's home to go to work or to school or to handle parenting tasks such as driving children to school and activities. Loss of occupations which may remind the victim of the trauma.

3. Inability to recall an important aspect of the trauma.

Possible Vocational Impairment: Suppression of the creative impulse. Survivor may have stopped painting, singing, dancing, writing. Loss of confidence. Suppression of the willingness to take the risk of new learning and challenge.

4. Markedly diminished interest in significant activities.

Possible Vocational Impairment: No interest in planning for the future. Difficulty in making commitments or in completion of education, classes, projects.

5. Feeling of detachment or estrangement from others.

Possible Vocational Impairment: Damage to social skills needed for interaction in educational and work settings. Damage to parenting skills.

6. Restricted range of affect (e.g., unable to have loving feelings).

Possible Vocational Impairment: Damage to social skills needed for interaction in work, school, and in the family. Suppression of pleasure, joy, and creativity in the activities of school, work, and home.

7. Sense of a foreshortened future (e.g. does not expect to have a career, marriage, or children, or a long life).

Possible Vocational Impairment: Difficulty in completing education including classes and degrees. Difficulty in keeping commitments including being on time, or keeping promises. Career and life planning efforts appear useless or impossible. May hold a deep seated belief that one is going to die soon, so why bother? The victim may not know that she holds this belief, but acts out of it anyway.

D.

Persistent symptoms of increased arousal (not present before the trauma), as indicated by two or more of the following:

1. Difficulty falling or staying asleep.

Possible Vocational Impairment: Lack of rest leading to lack of mental clarity on the job, in parenting, in classes. Fatigue leading to on the job injury or other accidents.

2. Irritability or outbursts of anger.

Possible Vocational Impairment: Difficulty in interactions with others, particularly supervisors or subordinates. Damage to parenting skills.

3. Difficulty concentrating.

Possible Vocational Impairment: Difficulty learning new tasks, performing complex and/or detailed tasks. Lack of self-confidence.

4. Hypervigiliance

Possible Vocational Impairment: Damage to social skills. Difficulty in risk taking, either no risks taken or the risk taking is inappropriate.

5. Exaggerated startle response.

Possible Vocational Impairment: Damage to social interactions. Fear of others. Fatigue.

E.

Duration of the disturbance (symptoms in B, C and D) is more than one month.

F.

The disturbance causes clinically significant distress or impairment in social, occupational, or other important areas of functioning.

Vocational Impairment Commentary written by Patricia A. Murphy, Ph.D., Diplomate, American Board of Vocational Experts, Certified Rehabilitation Counselor.

Vocational Impairment Commentary on CPTSD Diagnostic Criteria

> **COMPLEX POST-TRAUMATIC STRESS DISORDER**
>
> (The complex post-traumatic stress disorder diagnostic criteria is quoted from Judith Lewis Herman (1992, p. 121) in *Trauma and Recovery*).

1. A history of subjection to totalitarian control over a prolonged period (months to years). Examples include hostages, prisoners of war, concentration camp survivors, and survivors of some religious cults. Examples also include those subjected to totalitarian systems in sexual and domestic life, including survivors of domestic battering, childhood physical or sexual abuse, and organized sexual exploitation.

Possible Vocational Impairment: Long absences from the waged labor market, underemployment, inability to complete or continue educational and vocational preparation, criminal record (for being used in prostitution, welfare fraud), economic deprivation (homelessness, signing over all assets), l act of external support systems, loss of social skills, physical injuries (e.g., orthopedic injuries, closed head injury, dental trauma), chronic illnesses (malnutrition, pelvic diseases, substance abuse), chronic pain syndrome, chronic fatigue.

2. Alterations in affect regulation, including persistent dysphoria, chronic suicidal preoccupation, self- injury, explosive or extremely inhibited anger (may alternate), compulsive or extremely inhibited sexuality (may alternate).

Possible Vocational Impairment: Damage to social skills (e.g., difficulty with supervision and feedback in the workplace or at school), chronic health problems including substance abuse leading to absenteeism and poor performance in school and on the job, vulnerability to inducement and/or extortion into prostitution, vulnerability to sexual harassment on the job/in education).

3. Alterations in consciousness, including amnesia or hypermnesia for traumatic events, transient dissociative episodes, depersonalization/derealization, reliving experiences, either in the form of intrusive post-traumatic stress disorder symptoms or in the form of ruminative preoccupation.

Possible Vocational Impairment: Difficulty concentrating on tasks, new learning in the workplace and at school, delay and/or damage to developmental skills such as reading, language development, mathematics, possible lack of work identity, stunting of the creative process.

5. Alterations in perception of perpetrator, including preoccupation with relationship with perpetrator (includes preoccupation with revenge), unrealistic attribution of total power to perpetrator (caution: victim's assessment of power realities may be more realistic than clinician's), idealization or paradoxical gratitude, sense of special or supernatural relationship, acceptance of belief system or rationalizations of perpetrator.

Possible Vocational Impairment: May move with or follow perpetrator from city to city (e.g., in a marriage or in a pimp/prostitute relationship) which disrupts education and career development, escaping from perpetrator by going underground which also disrupts education and career, allow unwaged work skills (parenting/caretaking) to be degraded (e.g., children are abused in the name of discipline or perpetrator's special needs), accepts perpetrator's evaluation of the value of education, work, and money including the idea that having a higher level of skills, knowledge, education, work, and money than the perpetrator is a betrayal of the perpetrator, accepts perpetrator's control of money and the right to communicate with others, and holds these beliefs even if the perpetrator is dead.

6. Alterations in relations with others, including isolation and withdrawal, disruption in intimate relationships, repeated search for rescuer (may alternate with isolation and withdrawal), persistent distrust, repeated failures of self-protection.

Possible Vocational Impairment: Loss of support systems which would allow risk taking in career development, inappropriate relationships with teachers/mentors/bosses including sexual relationships and vulnerability to sexual harassment in the workplace and in the educational process, vulnerability to inducement into prostitution (average age of entry in the U.S. is between 13 and 16 years leading to further trauma and possible life long vocational impairment), inability to utilize mentoring or networking support in career development, underemployment by working in jobs which will insure isolation (e.g., working alone as a maid when the victim is a college graduate).

7. Alterations in systems of meaning including loss of sustaining faith, sense of hopelessness and despair.

Possible Vocational Impairment: No planning for the future, difficulty completing education and long range projects, no pleasure in work, lack of passion in all endeavors, suppression of the creative impulse, no sense of the value of contribution to be made to others, expectation that work will be oppressive, routine, and without joy, expectation that others in the workplace will either be oppressive or isolating, neglects parenting/caretaking duties because of no belief in the worth of life for one's self and one's children.

Vocational Impairment Commentary written by Patricia A. Murphy, Ph.D., Diplomate, American Board of Vocational Experts, Certified Rehabilitation Counselor.

four

---

reclaiming my innocent body

This book is dedicated with tenderness and respect to the blameless vulva.

Alice Walker, 1992

This chapter is dedicated with tenderness and respect to the blameless, innocent female body, your female body.

Alice Walker's ironically titled novel, *Possessing the Secret of Joy,* is an exploration of genital mutilation.

It is estimated that from ninety to one hundred million women and girls living today in Africa, Far Eastern, and Middle Eastern countries have suffered some form of genital mutilation.

Walker, 1992, p. 283

But it is not only women of Africa, the Far East, and Middle Eastern countries whose genitals are assaulted. The American co-researchers in *Making the Connections: Women, Work & Abuse* report venereal disease, sterilization, numbing below the waist, pain in the lower back/pelvis area, rape after cervical surgery, yeast infections, IUD perforation of the uterus, and hints of assaults and injuries to the genitals as just *some* of the physical injuries and diseases resulting from their abuse experiences. Walker takes the title of her novel from "a white colonialist author who has lived all her life among Africans and failed to see them as human beings who can be destroyed by suffering." This (fictional?) author wrote, "Black people are natural...they possess the secret of joy, which is why they can survive the suffering and humiliation inflicted upon them" (p. 271). Walker concludes her powerful novel with a protest. The male and female characters in her novel come together. They hold up a banner written in enormous letters, "**RESISTANCE IS THE SECRET OF JOY!**"

Reclaiming your innocent, blameless female body is an act of resistance. The purpose of this chapter is to increase your resistance to the power of denial which demands that you ignore or numb your body to the injuries inflicted upon it.

This denial is complex, pervasive, external, also sometimes self-imposed, and serves to support the notion that women and girls are not injured by rape, battering, incest, being used in prostitution by several men each day and night, or by the humiliation of verbal-emotional abuse of a hostile, harassing work environment. By ignoring the injuries to our bodies, we find ourselves blamed for our own abuse. This is because when the body is "disappeared" from the abuse story, the story becomes psychological only, and we are then thrust back to the culturally embedded character assassination of the trauma survivor, who is said to be lying, fantasizing, exaggerating.

This disappearance of the body from the story of traumatic abuse is never more ironic than when a battered woman goes to the emergency room. Studies indicate that "while 40% of all injuries presented by women occur in abusive relationships and 19% of female trauma patients are abused, abuse and battering are rarely identified (Kurz and Stark, 1988)." When a domestic violence survivor and I reviewed her emergency room records together in preparation for her domestic tort case, we discovered that her abuse injuries were not even noted in the records even though her injuries were quite visible. She was bleeding from her mouth where her teeth were showing through her lower lip. She had cuts and bruises on her face, her left eye, her legs and arms. Her shirt was bloodied. She received no treatment for her injuries whatsoever. Instead, she was treated for the conditions and symptoms defined by her battering husband, not the treating physician. The perpetrator said she was a suicidal, drug and alcohol abusing woman who needed to be referred to mental health. This is what the emergency room records document, and this is what the studies of emergency room treatment of battered women reveal. The battered woman's injuries are further obliterated by a process defined as "labeling."

> *Labeling is here specified as the act of designating behaviors, complaints, or groups in ways that seem devoid of therapeutic intent, that are unsupported by hard evidence, and through which providers can relieve their frustration by punitively blaming women for their problems.* (Kurz and Stark, 1988)

This situation had become so problematic that the American Medical Association finally developed guidelines for emergency room physicians at their national convention in 1992. The U.S. Surgeon General in 1992, Antonia Novello, noted that "domestic violence is rampant and doctors are part of the problem (Smolowe, 1992)."

So if it seems peculiar to include a chapter titled *Reclaiming My Innocent Body* in the section which is all about words (*I. The Tools — Gathering the Words of Power*), consider that it is with words that the female body is disappeared from emergency room records. It is with words that physically injured women are labeled as mentally ill, alcoholic, drug abusers, difficult, uncooperative. It is with words, definitions of disability, that we gain entry into benefit systems such Social Security Disability, workers' compensation, state departments of rehabilitation. It is with words that attorneys file domestic tort cases, civil incest, and sexual assault cases.

And it is with words that we reclaim our bodies by naming and defining the trauma as physical, as well as psychological, spiritual, soul-wrecking.

And if it seems peculiar to start this chapter with the stories of genital mutilation, consider that there is a link between women's sexuality and women's work. Vocational rehabilitation counselors accept as a truism that when a man is injured on his job and loses his work, his sexual functioning is often impaired. It seems that a man's work identity coexists with his sexual potency. (In my experience as a rehabilitationist in the California and Nevada workers' compensation systems, this may be more true for white men than men of color, who have been excluded from meaningful work by racism. This may mean, for men of color, the sense of self is not so tied to one's work status.)

How women's sexual functioning coexists with women's waged and unwaged work lives is not clear. The major hue and cry in most research on women and work is still centered on the problems middle class white women have raising their children while also working for wages. This, of course, leaves out everybody else who has always had to work for wages and raise her children at the same time, and perhaps raise the white woman's children, as well as her own. This research also excludes women who choose not to have children, or whose children are grown and gone. The differences between the career-focused middle class white woman and the career-focused middle class African American woman, or the Puerto Rican woman working as a maid, or as a college professor, has been rarely addressed in the vocational rehabilitation profession, or by career psychologists. Lesbian women of any color have also been excluded from such an analysis.

In my opinion, it is Black women who have contributed the most to an emerging theory of the connections between work, sexuality, and self for women. Black women have always had to deal with the issues of their sexuality, motherhood, and work (or slavery) simultaneously. To set the middle class white woman's experience of sexuality, motherhood, and work as the experience to be explored is to ignore the leadership, the contributions, and the *advanced* thinking of Black women scholars, writers, intellectuals, community leaders, and feminists. The depth and complexity of Black feminist thought on these issues cannot be addressed here in any detail, but Patricia Hill Collins' (1991) book, *Black Feminist Thought: Knowledge, Consciousness, and the Politics of Empowerment*, is important reading for all women, if for only the chapters, "Work, Family, and Black Women's Oppression" and "The Power of Self Definition."

Audre Lorde's essay in *Sister Outsider* (1984), *"The Uses of the Erotic"* teaches us all how "the power of the erotic within our lives can give us the energy to pursue genuine change within our world." Lorde's essay gives me the confidence to evolve a theory of genital celebration as the basis for the healing of women's work lives. I don't think it is an accident that such an idea, genital celebration, should evolve from the writing of Black women in general, and a Black lesbian-feminist (Audre Lorde) in particular (Lesbians, after all, are, or should be, the greatest celebrants of the vulva). And I don't think it is an accident that my beginnings of an understanding about all this took place when one of the vice-chancellors at the University of California at Santa Barbara brought an honored guest of the University to the

Women's Center, introducing her to me as a physician from Tunisia who performed clitoridectomies. As we stood there—brown woman, white woman, white man – I knew that my career at the University had been destroyed at the cruel intersection of sexism and racism. As a representative of the University, I had obligations to a guest. As a woman, I was bonded to the other woman in this triangle. As a white woman, I had the obligation to understand the consequences of my skin privilege. As a member of a colonialist country, I had to consider cultural imperialism. As a feminist, I was and am unalterably opposed to clitoridectomies. My leadership, my vision for the Women's Center were all smashed at that moment. I understood I was being punished for speaking out about a culture of rape during the terrible winter of 1977-78 when three young women fell victim to a serial murderer in the Santa Barbara area. In short, my academic career had been destroyed because my creativity had been mutilated, my erotic power disenfranchised.

This, then, is my theory. Creativity is the key. An assault on sexuality is an assault on creativity. A damaged creative impulse means a damaged work identity. A damaged work identity means injury to creativity, and injury to sexuality. Creativity, sexuality, and work identity all exist together. They are not separate. I don't think women and men are so different in this. I think we just know more about men's work, men's creativity, and men's sexuality than we do about women's. As I pointed out in *Making the Connections: Women, Work & Abuse*, in patriarchal society, a woman's identity as a worker is still not acknowledged, and her creativity is still relegated to her reproductive function. I think class, race, age, (dis)ability, and sexual preference add endless permutations to this theory much like a prism, which is dependent upon the quality of light poured into it. Or dependent upon what Collins (1991, pp. 11-13) would describe as an "angle of vision," when we look through it. One way to tell if a feminist theory is on the right track is by the reaction of the patriarchy. The explosive and negative reaction to Judy Chicago's *The Dinner Party Project* by the House of Representatives in 1990 indicates to me that the intimate linkages among creativity, sexuality, and work or achievement are real (Lippard, 1990). (Chicago's *Dinner Party* is extensively explored in the next section of the Workbook, *Section II. The Process — Moving Through The Flower.*) This massive artwork is a symbolic history of the achievements of women in Western Civilization. Thirty-nine of the women are represented by place settings made of china-painted ceramic plates and needleworked runners or tablecloths for each setting. The plates are executed with a butterfly or vaginal motif. Chicago illuminates the linkages between women's sexuality, creativity, and achievement (or work) in these controversial sculptures. Her work was called "clearly pornographic" by Representative Stan Parris.

Art critic Lucy Lippard (1990) notes that "the Congress's over-zealous amateur art critics never did pick up on the total form of Chicago's piece: the inverted triangle, an ancient symbol of female power, also derives from the dread genital region." And as Chicago herself has demanded, "If towers, spires, thrusting sculptural forms and aggressive shapes can be discussed in terms of their esthetic, rather than their phallic implications, why can't open, metamorphosing forms be understood in terms of their multilayered beauty?" (Lippard, 1990).

Alice Walker also had a negative reaction to *The Dinner Party*, but not because of the vaginal imagery. Her complaint is that Sojourner Truth is represented with three faces and not a vagina. Walker writes, "Better then to deny that the black woman has a vagina. Is capable of motherhood. Is a woman" (Walker, 1980, p. 131).

In this workbook, Walker and Chicago, are brought together to celebrate the female body, the vagina—Chicago with *The Dinner Party*, and Walker with her beautiful words:

> *A vagina the color of raspberries and blackberries—or scupper-nongs and muscadines—and of that strong, silvery sweetness, with as well a sharp flavor of salt.*
>
> *Walker, 1980, pp. 131-132*

With the help of these two women, we reclaim our sexuality, our body's creativity, because without access to our creativity we cannot reach our full vocational potential — in our work with our children, or in our work in the world for wages, or both. Genital mutilation is the most specific expression of the assault on women's creativity and sexuality, but all assaults on women and girls resulting in any injury or disease are also assaults on women's sexuality, creativity, and their work lives. Genital celebration, by contrast, is the most specific expression of our creativity, our sexuality, our achievement. Genital celebration is also a form of resistance, and resistance, as we have learned, is the secret of joy.

the physical injuries and inflicted diseases of abuse survivors

> *What they recorded was the mechanism of injury...*
> Carole Warshaw, 1993

The denial of injury/disease inflicted upon abuse survivors also became apparent when I attempted to discover research which would give us an overview of the major injuries and disease processes of abuse survivors. *The Journal of the American Medical Association* devoted its June 17, 1992 issue to domestic violence. I pounced on the article, *Assessing for Abuse During Pregnancy: Severity and Frequency of Injuries and Associated Entry Into Prenatal Care*, with mixed feelings. First, I thought, "Good, I'll find a chart, a list, a paragraph describing the injuries." My next thought was that this information had been developed for pregnant women only and not for all those other times (most of our life spans in the United States) when we are not pregnant. I humphed in disapproval while muttering over women, work, and abuse issues, and the complications of adding pregnant working women to the mix. Imagine my dismay when I discovered that Table 3 listed the frequency of the abuse, the perpetrator of the abuse, and mashed descriptions of *abusive behaviors* (slapping, pushing, punching) in with descriptions of *abuse injuries* (head injury, internal injury, wound from weapon) (McFarlane, Parker, Soeken, & Bullock, 1992).

This is very odd. When describing injuries sustained in an automobile accident, I don't think we care if the steering wheel or the door handle punctured the survivor's lung. We leave such descriptions to the police or the attorneys who may need to write an accident report or a legal brief in a personal injury case. Medical descriptions of battering which focus on the battering instead of the injury to the victim are another way to obliterate the reality of the victim's experience, to deny the pain and suffering she experiences in her body and to deny her the reality of her body. (This is not in any way meant to suggest that the cause of the survivor's injury(ies) should be ignored.) To confuse and blur abusive behaviors with abuse injuries is to focus on the perpetrator. Once again, the survivor is rendered invisible.

overcoming invisibility – conscious breathing as resistance

Also, breath connected me to my body. Whether my mind wandered or not, my body stayed in the cross-legged position. It was here, whether I was or not.

Natalie Goldberg, 1993

Most abuse survivors are highly skilled at leaving their bodies, of not being present. One way to resist the pervasive denial of your body by society in general, and the medical profession in particular, is to stay present in your own body. And one very simple way to do this is to breathe consciously, easily, and deeply. If you find that you have split or disassociated, when you become aware that you have been absent, breathe. If you know that you are about to leave your body, breathe. As you become a skilled conscious breather, you will become aware of when you are holding your breath. This awareness will empower you for further conscious breathing, and signal you that you are about to be rendered invisible by someone (maybe yourself) or something. Your body has a knowingness which is your birthright, and your breath is the messenger of your body's knowledge. Breathing is socially acceptable, and can be done anywhere — the courtroom, the emergency room, at the doctor's, with your rehabilitation counselor, your therapist, your recovery group, at school, on the job. Breathing is life itself, and your breathing is both celebration and resistance.

> **TIP**
> If reading any of the material in this chapter or in any part of the Workbook causes you to "disappear," feel frightened, or overwhelmed, taking at least three deep, slow, and lazy breaths will help. You also have the power to direct your breath to parts of your body if you are feeling numbness, pain or sensations in your body which are disturbing to you. Close your eyes, breathe, think the breath into your whole body or parts of your body.

RESOURCE – The chapter titled, "Your Body" in *The Courage to Heal: A Guide for Women Survivors of Child Sexual Abuse* by Ellen Bass and Laura Davis is also valuable for survivors of battering, rape, sexual harassment, ritual abuse, and the prostitution trauma.

overcoming invisibility – naming the physical injury(ies)/inflicted diseases to my innocent body

There is a closet in my hallway here that, of course, has a door handle on it. I backed up against it, and it hits me right at the spot the X-ray showed... I just slid down the wall and cried. To realize how I'd kept that pain pretty much to myself. So from head to tailbone the man destroyed my spine, broke bones in my hands and feet and ribs, and may have caused some brain damage.

Colleen S. Gibbons, June 6, 1993

Although we are still in the beginning stages of documenting the physical injury and disease which result from abuse, every researcher or writer on abuse reports injury and disease as one of the consequences of abuse. Every system of the body is involved (Koss & Heslet, September, 1992). This is true if we are examining the consequences of rape (Koss & Heslet, September, 1992, Warshaw, 1988, pp. 71-73), woman battering (American Medical Association, 1992, Murphy, 1993, pp. 69-77, Walker, 1979, pp. 223-225, Warshaw, 1993), sexual harassment (Evans, 1978), child sexual abuse (Bass & Davis, 1988, pp. 207-222, 446-457), child battering (Kempe, Silverman, Steele, Droegemueller, & Silver, 1982), and sexual exploitation in prostitution (Murphy, 1993, pp. 69-77, Neland, undated).

The purpose of this section is to assist you in identifying injury and disease which may have been caused by your traumatic abuse experience(s), and to pinpoint how that injury or disease may have damaged your vocational potential in the waged work world and your unwaged working capacities with your children, your home-making duties. The *Overcoming Invisibility – Reclaiming My Innocent Body Exercises* are divided into three sections. The first section reflects the acute or immediate consequences of the traumatic experience, and the second section addresses the chronic or long-lasting effects of the traumatic experience(s). The third section involves the catastrophic results of traumatic abuse leading to disability and the abuse of women with preexisting disabling conditions. The exercises are based on the frequently noted injuries/diseases by the researchers and writers listed above. A complete listing of all injuries and diseases is beyond the scope of this Workbook.

RESOURCE – *A Guide to Rehabilitation* by Paul M. Deutsch and Horace W. Sawyer is a two-volume work which lists injuries, diseases, treatments, vocational impairments, and vocational outcomes. Published by Ahab Press, Inc., this excellent resource can be located in law libraries.

TIP

The insertion of dates of injuries in the exercises is meant to be a helpful tool for those of you who are planning to file a civil incest, sexual assault, or domestic tort lawsuit. The listing of the dates of injuries/inflicted diseases is also helpful in understanding the pattern of abuse and the subsequent pattern of your educational and vocational history (e.g., Dropping out of school after being raped. Losing a job after a beating. Having an arrest record for prostitution.)

OVERCOMING INVISIBILITY –
RECLAIMING MY INNOCENT BODY EXERCISES

I. THE IMMEDIATE CONSEQUENCES OF TRAUMATIC ABUSE

Bleeding Injuries (e.g., Wounds around face and head requiring stitches, gunshot wounds, knife wounds.) My bleeding injury(ies) can be described as:

_____

_____

_____

_____

This (these) injury(ies) took place on (approximate date): _____

Other bleeding injuries took place on (approximate date(s), and are described as:

_____

_____

_____

_____

Acute Vocational Impairment (e.g., This [these] bleeding injury[ies] meant that I took off work for a few days, made up stories and lies to tell my children and friends, laid in bed for three days, put pounds of makeup on so I could go out to work, back onto the streets.) What happened to me is:

_____

_____

_____

_____

Internal Injuries (e.g., Damaged spleens, kidneys, punctured lungs.) My internal injury(ies) were:

_____

_____

_____

_____

_____

And took place on (approximate date): _____

Other internal injuries were inflicted on (approximate date[s]): _____

and can be described as: _____

_____

_____

_____

_____

Acute Vocational Impairment (e.g., This [these] internal injuries meant that my work life [for wages and/or in my home] was disrupted as follows):

_____

_____

_____

_____

_____

_____

_____

Bones (e.g., Cracked vertebrae, ribs, skulls, pelvises, broken arms, hands, legs, jaws, collarbones). I had broken bones and fractures as follows:

_____

_____

_____

_____

This (these) injury(ies) were inflicted on (approximate) date: _____

Other injury(ies) to my (jaw, back, arms, legs) took place on (approximate dates):

_____

and can be described as follows: _____

_____

_____

_____

_____

Acute Vocational Impairment (e.g., I lost my job because the cracked vertebrae in my neck meant that I couldn't look down into a microscope. I took so many pain pills I had trouble concentrating at work. It was difficult for me to do housework and diaper the baby with my arm in a sling.) My experience was:

_____

_____

_____

_____

_____

_____

Burns (e.g., Cigarette burns, burns from irons, stoves, hot coffee.) My burns can be described as:

_____

_____

_____

_____

This (these) injury(ies) took place on (approximate date): _____

I have been burned other times (approximate dates): _____

These injuries are: _____

_____

_____

_____

_____

Acute Vocational Impairment (e.g., I was in so much pain that I had difficulty concentrating on my work duties. I took days off from work. I kept my eldest child home from school to help me.) My experience was that:

_____

_____

_____

_____

_____

_____

Invisible Injuries (e.g., Hyperventilation, anxiety attacks, abdominal pain, chemical dependency, chronic headaches, recurrent vaginal infections, depression, heart palpitations, crying spells, suicidal tendencies.) I have used the medical system to try to get help for my invisible injury(ies) which I would describe as follows:

_____

_____

_____

_____

_____

The last time I went to the doctor, the emergency room for this (these) problem(s) was (approximate date):_____. I've been to the doctor, the chiropractor, the emergency room for this (number of times) in the past year _____and I have been given the following medication for these symptoms:

_____

_____

_____

Acute Vocational Impairment (e.g., My headaches prevent me from working a steady job. I don't leave the house much because I'm so afraid. I'm too afraid to apply for a job, or get into school. I go to the doctor too much and I'm in trouble at work, school because of absenteeism and tardiness. My kids avoid me when I have one of my spells. I'm collecting pain pills and tranquilizers for when it gets really bad. My grades were really back in grade school/high school because I couldn't concentrate. I dropped out of school.) My invisible injuries have caused me to:

_____

_____

_____

_____

Genital Injuries (e.g., Vaginal and perineal lacerations and tears.) As a result of the acquaintance rape, stranger rape, marital rape, incest trauma, and/or battering, I have experienced the following injury(ies) to my genitals:

_____

_____

_____

_____

These injuries took place on (approximate date)_____. I have had prior experience of this kind of injury which are described as:

_____

_____

_____

_____

and occurred on (approximate dates)_____.

Acute Vocational Impairment (e.g., I felt so much shame, I couldn't leave my apartment for days. I had so much pain and bleeding I had to stay home and miss work/school. I missed a job interview, a trip to Europe. I was unable to participate in Girl Scout activities. I had to go to the bathroom when no one else was around at school/at work. I felt really ugly. I stopped painting/music/writing. I turned my first trick a few days/weeks later.) My experience was that I:

_____

_____

_____

_____

Sexually Transmitted Diseases (e.g., I contracted gonorrhea, syphilis, chlamydia, hepatitis B, HIV/AIDS, herpes. I developed pelvic inflammatory disease because of untreated STD.) I was told I had:

_____

_____

_____

on (approximate date)_____. Because my STD was untreated for so long, I also developed the following complications:

_____

_____

_____

_____

_____

Acute Vocational Impairment (e.g., I was too embarrassed to use my health insurance through work and so I had to use my educational fund savings to treat my STD. I had so much pain from pelvic inflammatory disease I missed many days of work, and had trouble paying attention on the job.) What I experienced is:

_____

_____

_____

_____

_____

_____

Pregnancy (e.g., I was one of the 5% of rape victims who became pregnant. My father impregnated me. My husband did not allow me to use birth control. When I was pregnant, my husband punched my stomach more than he did before. The battering increased after I got pregnant. I lost my baby after a beating. After I got pregnant, my pimp forced me into increasingly violent pornography.) My experience of pregnancy was:

_____

_____

_____

This happened (approximate date)_____.

I have had other experiences with abuse and pregnancy: _____

_____

_____

_____

_____

These experiences took place on (approximate dates)_____.

Acute Vocational Impairment (e.g., I dropped out of grade school/high school/college because of my pregnancy. I lost a good job. I went on sick leave. I was unable to do much for my children while I was recovering. I have lost one of my dreams in life, which was to be a mother. I now have a child to care for I didn't want.) The damage to my waged and unwaged work life is:

_____

_____

_____

_____

_____

II. THE LONG TERM CONSEQUENCES OF TRAUMATIC ABUSE

Chronic Pain Syndromes (e.g., I experience pelvic pain, and I have experienced various medical interventions and procedures as a result. I have had a terrible time since my hysterectomy. I have pain most of the time in my neck, mid-back, lower back, jaw, face. I grind my teeth at night. I've been diagnosed with TMJ. I have had chronic headaches since grade school.) My experience of chronic pain can be described as follows:

_____

_____

_____

_____

This pain started (approximate date) _____.

I have used the following medical procedures, hospitalizations, prescribed drugs, and nonprescription drugs (alcohol, marijuana) to try to get relief:

_____

_____

_____

_____

_____

Other chronic pain I experience is:

_____

_____

_____

_____

_____

This pain started on (approximate date) _____.

I have used various methods to handle it, including: _____

_____

_____

_____

_____

Chronic Vocational Impairment (e.g., I feel angry most of the time. I've given up trying to work. I can no longer work as a waitress, nurse, in child care, as a secretary. I can't sit through a class in the classrooms at the college. I can't do stock work anymore. I've been on disability forever. I got hurt again on the job, and now I'm on workers' compensation. My husband, my partner has to do most of the housework. My kids do the cooking. I feel ashamed that I'm not a good parent. I can't get ahead because I spend too much money on managing my pain by buying muscle relaxants and going to the chiropractor.) My experience of chronic pain and my work is:

_____

_____

_____

_____

_____

_____

_____

_____

_____

_____

Premenstrual Syndrome (e.g., I have PMS, and I've gone to great lengths to handle it.) My experience is that:

_____

_____

_____

_____

_____

_____

My PMS started (approximate date or age of onset)_____.

Chronic Vocational Impairment (e.g., This has meant that I spent a day in per month all through high school, and I still miss lots of work. I scream at my kids. I get drunk. I overeat. Then I don't want to do anything. Its hard to focus when I'm having PMS.) What happens to me in my waged and unwaged work life during my monthly PMS is:

_____

_____

_____

_____

_____

_____

_____

_____

_____

_____

Gastrointestinal Symptoms (e.g., I've been diagnosed with irritable bowel syndrome, non-ulcer dyspepsia, chronic abdominal pain. I experience diarrhea and/or constipation frequently. I have these problems along with chronic pelvic pain for a long time.) My experience has been:

_____

_____

_____

_____

_____

_____

This all started (approximate date of onset)_____.

Chronic Vocational Impairment (e.g., When I get scared, I get diarrhea. This means it's hard for me to take test in school or for a job. The pain distracts me from paying attention to my work, to my kids. I can only eat at home which means I've never been to the company picnic.) My experience of how my gastrointestinal symptoms has changed my work life at school/on the job and at home is:

_____

_____

_____

_____

_____

_____

_____

_____

_____

Unhealthy Behaviors (e.g., I have an eating disorder — bulimia, anorexia. Substance abuse has been/is one of my problems. I never fasten my seat belt in the car. I have cut myself on the arms/legs. I don't care if I get HIV/AIDS.) Some negative health behaviors I have engaged in are:

_____

_____

_____

_____

_____

_____

_____

Chronic Vocational Impairment (e.g., I have lost jobs because of my substance abuse problems. I started turning tricks in order to support my drug habit. I dropped out of school. I lost my children because of my drug/alcohol problems. I can't get health insurance because I have HIV, and I can't get a job because of my prison record. I've lost my ability to read or learn. I started drinking when I was ten years old.) My education, work, life as a parent has been damaged in the following ways:

_____

_____

_____

_____

_____

_____

_____

III. CATASTROPHIC CONSEQUENCES OF ABUSE

Catastrophic Injuries Resulting from Traumatic Abuse (e.g., As a result of battering, rape, childhood assault, I became paraplegic. I have a traumatic brain injury. I lost my sight, my hearing. My arms were amputated. My throat was cut.) My experience of catastrophic injury is:

_____

_____

_____

_____

_____

This injury occurred on (date) _____.

Vocational Impairment (e.g., I lost my profession as a teacher, scholar, bus driver, artist. I lost years out of my educational endeavors. I lost my house, my husband. I can't have children. I have become dependent upon welfare, Social Security Disability Insurance. I am poor. I can't get health insurance. I can't get a job. I can't get a van, a computer, a better wheelchair. Vocational rehabilitation is a joke.) My work life, my unwaged work at home has changed in the following ways:

_____

_____

_____

_____

_____

_____

_____

Pre-existent Disability and Traumatic Abuse (e.g., Like many women with disabilities, I have experienced sexual and physical abuse. My physical health has deteriorated as a result. I am no longer able to do the things I could do before.) The combination of abuse and disability has had the following consequences in my daily life activities:

_____

_____

_____

_____

_____

_____

_____

Vocational Impairment (e.g., My fatigue levels mean that I no longer have the strength to fight to get a van, a computer, better equipment for myself. I am unable to sustain my part time job. I have had recurring infections since the abuse.) My experience of abuse has meant that the quality of my work life, my daily activities, my child care and home keeping duties have changed as follows:

_____

_____

_____

_____

_____

_____

TIP

Three deep and lazy breaths are recommended at this point in the Workbook. Facing the vulnerability of the body to traumatic abuse challenges us all on the deepest levels. Allow the cleansing power of your own breath to recall the power of the life flowing within you. The Hindus say that the moment between darkness and sunrise is when the whole world takes a breath, and as the song tells us, we are the world.

This chapter and the previous chapter, *Naming the Trauma*, have prepared us for using the affirmation process described in *Overcoming Verbal-Emotional Abuse*. It is not enough to identify the hurt to our bodies and minds although it is a necessary first step in the recovery process. In order to discover the secret of joy, we must learn the tools of resistance. We must transform the trauma, mental and physical, so that we get the best revenge of all — living well.

five

overcoming verbal-emotional abuse

Words were perceived as weapons. Words were used to separate and diminish people, not to connect and empower them. The silent women worried that they would be punished just for using words— any words.

Mary Field Belenky, Blythe McVicker Clinchy,
Nancy Rule Goldberger, and Jill Mattuck Tarule, 1986

The purpose of this part of the Workbook is to allow you take your power over words, to use words to connect with yourself and your needs and desires. And to empower yourself, your children, your loved ones. The exercises which follow are meant to be suggestions which will encourage you to discover the words and phrases which were used against you as weapons so that you may transform them into life-affirming language deep within your being. The previous chapters may have brought up intensely disturbing or negative thoughts. This chapter will enable you to transform those thoughts. You might even regard them as compost to be used to grow a new life.

getting started: a meditation

If this seems frightening to you, you may wish to engage in the following meditation. The purpose of the meditation is to create a safe and calm oasis inside yourself where the work of self-affirmation can take place. You may wish to light a candle, or burn some sweet grass, or use a smudge stick to purify the atmosphere. In the beginning stages of your self-affirmation work, you will need to find a place where you can have privacy and where you can either write or speak aloud into a tape recorder. Later you will find that you can evoke this sense of safety inside yourself easily and without the need for a special place just by breathing (e.g., I spent more than two years doing my self-affirmation work on the freeways while driving from my office to appointments all over the Los Angeles Basin).

Sit comfortably. Put both feet on the floor so that the strength of Mother Earth supports you fully. Rest your arms and hands easily with the palms up so that you are able to experience the flow of energy within your hands. Your hands are blessed. They are that part of your body which allows you to cook, to tend your baby, to touch in love, to paint, to type, to write, to create.

Close your eyes. Take three deep, slow breaths. Let the exhalation on these breaths be as slow and as lazy as the inhalations. Continue this lazy breathing. If you forget, it's not a problem. Just start the slow and lazy breathing again. Imagine the sounds of your breathing spreading throughout your body, making a sweet and peaceful silence. Imagine the fragrant air of your breath as light, and as a space opening into an oasis, your oasis. This might be a place of beauty and safety from your own life where you felt free and beautiful, or a dream you've had, or something you saw in a movie or read in a book, or it may be new, even a surprise to you now. Incorporate the sounds, the images, the smells from your surroundings into the sounds, the images, the smells from your inner oasis. The ticking of clock and the water lapping against a shoreline. The smell of cooking and the fragrance of pine needles. The rush of wind through tree tops and the voices of children playing outside your window. Let that be.

Notice your body. What are you feeling in your hands, your chest, your legs, your feet? Is your head heavy? Whatever you notice is just fine. Let it be.

Keep breathing in slow and easy inhalations and exhalations. Whatever comes up, remember you are safe now. Don't push away any image, thought, or feeling. Let it be. Keep breathing. The breath will move through your body and take the image, thought, or feeling. Stay with your breathing.

Allow your guide to appear in this place. Your guide may be a woman or a man, a child or an animal. If you don't see a guide, that's okay. You may call upon Artemis. She is a Greek Goddess who protects new life, all new life. She protects the new born, the very young. There is even an herb used during birthing named after her, Artemisia. She is very powerful. A hunter came into Her forest to kill one of Her deer. She transformed him into a deer with a flick of Her hand. She transformed him into the innocent being he once was. She will protect you too as you grow into your new life. The bear is also sacred to Artemis. So if a bear appears to you, it is probably Artemis in disguise. You are safe now. If your guide gives you a gift—a feeling, a plant, a smile—accept it. Let that be. Keep breathing slow and easy breaths. When you are ready, open your eyes.

If you feel comfortable with writing, you may wish to write about your meditation. If writing is something you do not wish to do, you may record your thoughts and feelings aloud into a tape recorder. You may wish to describe your oasis, your guide, your gift. If you don't have the words or if you did not see your oasis, your guide, your gift very clearly, you may wish to describe your feelings. You are safe now. If you choose to continue with this meditation in the days ahead, your perceptions will become clearer. If you had a memory of abuse, you may wish to record this memory so that you can share it with your therapist or in your recovery group. If you heard a negative thought or the sound of words used as weapons, record this either in writing or on tape. You will learn to transform these hurtful words into affirmations.

Now that you are calm and protected, you may choose to do some self affirmation work.

TIP

If you like, you may tape this meditation guidance onto an audio tape in your own voice to play back for yourself. This is an example of affirming and nurturing yourself. This meditation is a suggestion, not a command. For example, the Goddess Artemis may not be an appropriate guide for you. Spider Woman, the Virgin of Guadalupe, Kuan Yin, Mawu, Fuji, or some other Goddess might have more of a rightness for you. You may wish to create your own guided meditation. Explore *The Great Cosmic Mother: Rediscovering the Religion of the Earth* by Monica Sjoo and Barbara Mor, *Descent to the Goddess: A Way of Initiation for Women* by Sylvia Brinton Perera, *Ancient Mirrors of Womanhood: A Treasury of Goddess and Heroine Lore from Around the World* and *When God Was A Woman* by Merlin Stone, *Hindu Goddesses: Visions of the Divine Feminine in the Hindu Religious Tradition* by David Kinsley, and *Lost Goddesses of Early Greece: A Collection of Pre-Hellenic Mythology* by Charelene Spretnak.

TIP

If the guided meditation makes you uneasy for any reason, simply do the lazy, easy breathing. If at any point in doing the exercises in the Workbook you feel uneasy, breathe through it slowly and easily. Notice what's happening in your body at that time.

TIP

Remember The Three Laws of Recovery: Law #1: Sobriety is the first priority. Law #2: Trust your hesitations. Law #3: You decide (Neland, undated).

affirmations

We all talk to ourselves, mostly inside our heads in a life-long inner dialogue. We talk to other people and other people talk to us, and we talk about others and others talk about us. Affirmations rest upon these relationships which use the words *I, you,* and *she.* When we have been told over and over, *you're so stupid,* eventually we include those words within our inner dialogue, and we say, *I'm so stupid.* We may also hear our abuser saying to other people, *she's so stupid.* If this verbal-emotional abuse took place when we were very young or over a long period of time, we take it deep inside of ourselves as a belief. We may not even remember or know that we believe this about ourselves because, by now, we just take it for granted. We just assume, *I'm so stupid.* Then, we act out of that hidden but very deep belief. Some of us will be afraid to go to school or learn something new. Others will find themselves angry or intimidated by people they think are smarter or more educated than themselves. Verbal-emotional abuse or psychological maltreatment can have profound, injurious, and long-lasting effects. Affirmations are one way to overcome and heal the effects of verbal-emotional abuse.

Affirmations are particularly important in the process of vocational or career and life planning because new learning either in an educational setting or on the job is a stressful process. Vocational rehabilitation or the process of healing the impairment created by abuse to your vocational potential always involves risk and challenge. For example, you may need to move to another city for a job or education in a new field. The development of better parenting skills may mean challenging the ideas and rules your parents gave you. Managing and earning your own money may lead you to confront not only your ideas about the role of women in society, but the ideas of others about who and what women are supposed to be. Just the act of signing up for a class at your local community college may bring you into direct conflict with your hidden belief system (*I'm so stupid. What makes me think I can learn anything?*), and your perpetrator's words as weapons (*You're so stupid. What makes you think you can learn anything?*). If you find yourself within a rehabilitation system such as workers' compensation or using the services of the state department of rehabilitation, you may find yourself intimidated and even angry with the counselors and other professionals. This is because your deeply buried idea about yourself as stupid will be forming the basis for your responses to these professionals. This does not put you in the best position to manage your own rehabilitation and vocational planning.

how to create affirmations out of words used as weapons

The basic tasks of self-affirmation work are identification, transformation, and repetition. Identification involves the process of discovering the negative thoughts and beliefs we hold about ourselves. Transformation is the process of turning the negative thoughts and beliefs into affirmations. Repetition of the affirmations is the healing process which can be tailor made to suit your personal preferences, and your life circumstances.

identification

Most of us have one deep core thought or belief about ourselves around which many or most of our other negative thoughts and beliefs cluster. In my case, the thought was *I, Pat am a bad person.* A thought like this is something you tell yourself in the dead of the night when everything is quiet. This small, still and terrible voice is your belief that what your abuser has told you is true. It is important to discover the core thought because it is the most powerful, and because it's transformation into its opposite *(I, Pat am innocent, and I forgive myself completely),* will also transform many or most of the other negative thoughts which stick to the core thought like so many flies on flypaper. In my case, this deep seated belief also led to such negative beliefs that I did not deserve love or money or comfort or any of the good things in life.

I did not discover nor understand that this was my core negative belief about myself until I had gained some experience with self-affirmation work with others in a group recovery experience. A guide emerged from this group. It was almost as though she had manifested herself from a meditation. I can see her beautiful lined face now, her white hair, her brightly painted hoop earrings, her face illuminated with kindness. This old woman listened to my story of abuse, turned to me, and announced the affirmation which was to reveal my inner core belief, *You, Pat are innocent, and you forgive yourself completely.* Her gift has stayed with me all these years, and given me a profound faith in the crone aspect of the experience of womanhood.

> **TIP**
> The process of identifying negative thoughts and feelings, of writing down or tapping hurtful and insulting words and phrases used by your abuser(s) may feel uncomfortable or lead to a sensation of numbness both emotionally and in your body. You may wish to use the meditation and/or the slow and lazy breathing described under *Getting Started: A Meditation.*

When the Sacred Crone gave me the gift of this affirmation, I was finally able to reach past a layer of ice over a deep pool of tears and sadness. I felt as though my heart had melted. My response was emotional, physical, and intellectual from the first moment. Once I understood that this was the core affirmation I needed, I then used it as the opening affirmation in my repetition exercises because this affirmation meant that all the following affirmations became more powerful since they were based in my reality.

You may understand what your core negative belief is immediately, or you may need to do some self-affirmation work for awhile before you can discover it. Either way is correct. Your core negative belief is unique to you. Your core affirmation will be uniquely yours as well. Whatever the negative belief is, it is usually very simple and very profound. That is, you do not want to use complicated language in either identifying negative thoughts or in creating their affirmations. This is because our inner dialogue with ourselves does not use complicated language such as: *You, Pat are a morally reprehensible individual.* The small, still and terrible voice is simple and devastating: *You, Pat are a bad person.* As a child, I probably said to myself: *You, Patty are a bad girl.*

You may not be so fortunate as to have a crone with hoop earrings and white hair to give you the gift of your core negative belief and its transformation in one mo-

> **TIP**
> Forgiveness is a complex issue, but it is my opinion that unless you can forgive yourself, your healing is not complete. This is not to imply that you are or have been at fault in any way. However, my own experience is that I blamed myself for my abuse, and so I needed to forgive myself. I don't think my experience of self-blame is unusual. Further, I do not hold the belief that forgiveness of the abuser is necessary for healing. To put it another way, forgiveness of yourself is the core forgiveness. It may be that the forgiveness of others will follow, but this is not a goal.

ment, but the work in the previous chapters may give you a place to start. Some clues to striking gold could include a sensation of profound numbness, a sense of emptiness and distance; tears welling up; bodily responses such as headache, stomach, or tension in the shoulders; any strong feelings of rage, hate, even laughter; leaving your body; slipping into another personality.

One simple place to start is to make a list of the words, phrases, and sentences you remember your abuser using.

My List of Words, Phrases, or Sentences As Weapons

(e.g., *You can't do anything right! You'll go to hell for that! Honor your father and mother. Who do you think you are? You're so stupid. The older you get, the dumber you get. Look at me when I talk to you.*)

_____

_____

_____

_____

_____

_____

_____

_____

_____

_____

_____

_____

_____

_____

_____

_____

Are There Words, Phrases, or Sentences Which Seem to Belong Together?

(e.g., *You'll go to hell for that, Honor your father and mother, Who do you think you are?* and *Can't you do anything right?, Look at me when I talk to you* all seem to cluster around negative thoughts which have to do with not being a good person. The remainder of the thoughts appear to center on competence – *you're so stupid and The older you get, the dumber you get.*)

Put the negative thoughts which belong together into clusters.

Cluster #1: _____

_____

_____

_____

Cluster #2: _____

_____

_____

_____

Cluster #3: _____

_____

_____

_____

Cluster #4: _____

_____

_____

_____

> **TIP**
>
> Feel free to add clusters on another piece of paper. You may or may not end up with four or more clusters. Any number is the right number.

Now reduce each Cluster into one simple negative thought.

(e.g. *I, Pat am a bad person* or *I, Patty am a bad person* for Cluster #1. Cluster #2 can be reduced to *I, Pat am stupid*.)

Simple Negative Thought #1: _____

Simple Negative Thought #2: _____

Simple Negative Thought #3: _____

Simple Negative Thought #4: _____

> **TIP**
>
> The reduction of a cluster of negative thoughts into one simple negative thought allows you to create the most powerful corresponding affirmation while keeping you from the dreary task of having to create an affirmation for every single word, phrase or sentence used against you as a weapon. Best of all, a single affirmation created for a cluster of these nasty words as weapons will transform the whole group.

transformation

When we discover an insulting comment, a hurtful name, a negative thought or belief we hold about ourselves, we have the power to transform that comment, hurtful name, negative thought or belief into an affirmation by simply changing it into its opposite. For example, *I'm so stupid* now becomes *I am intelligent*. To make this affirmation even more powerful, add your own name after *I* as in *I, Pat am intelligent*. If the verbal-emotional assault took place when you were a child and you had a child name, use that name as in *I, Patty am intelligent*.

> **TIP**
> If you were told over and over that you were stupid (or whatever hurtful thing was said to you) in a language other than English, it is important to create affirmations in the language of the abusive words. The affirmation is then more specific to the verbal-emotional assault, and therefore a more powerful affirmation.

> **TIP**
> If you feel overwhelmed by negative thoughts, see *Getting Started: A Meditation*. You may wish to use this meditation prior to doing your self-affirmation work. Feeling overwhelmed may also be a signal to see a therapist or go to a recovery group.

If you can't remember the words used as weapons against you (because you've blocked them out) or just because you're having a hard time getting started, refer to the previous chapters. Working the exercises in the previous chapters will most likely bring back some negative thoughts. You may wish to use the space provided to make your own lists. Recording both the negative thoughts and the affirmations are important for abuse survivors because one of our survival techniques is to block out, to "forget" the hurtful things said or done to us. To make a record is allow ourselves to move into healing since we no longer need to practice denial in order to survive.

> **TIP**
> In fact, it is good practice to thank ourselves for "forgetting." Because the "forgetting" worked. We survived, but now this technique is no longer useful. It is time to say thank you to ourselves, and move on.

> **TIP**
> An affirmation should not have negatives in it because our minds just dismiss the negatives, and you may end up with the opposite of what you want. For example, *I, Pat am not a bad person* turns itself into *I, Pat am a bad person*. Affirmations should be stated positively as in *I, Pat, am a good and lovable person* or *I, Pat am innocent and I forgive myself completely*.

Now transform the simple negative thought or thoughts you have selected into their opposites, the affirmations. *(e.g., I, Patty am a bad girl becomes I, Patty am innocent and I forgive myself completely. I, Pat am stupid becomes I, Pat, am intelligent.)*

Affirmation #1: _____

Affirmation #2: _____

Affirmation #3: _____

Affirmation #4: _____

Congratulations! You now have affirmations to use as tools in your recovery. You now know how to transform words as weapons into healing tools. This means that you may create an affirmation anytime you need one for a particular situation in your life as well as having a set of affirmations for healing the deep, inner hurt. The next step is the use of your affirmations.

repetition

Repetition is the method for using the affirmations you have just created. The repetition of the affirmations heals the deep, inner negative beliefs you hold about yourself. After all, it was the repetition of words, phrases, and sentences which created your deep negative beliefs in the first place. Affirmations used in this way are so powerful that they will heal years of repeated verbal emotional abuse in a short period of time. The time will vary from person to person. I spent more than two years with my set of affirmations which I repeated at least five days per week. When compared to my experience of at least 18 years of verbal-emotional abuse and all the succeeding years in which I cemented these beliefs deep inside myself, this was a brief time indeed. Now I use my affirmations on an as needed basis.

Happily, the benefits are immediate. Once you have started your self-affirmation work you will notice that you will have increased self-awareness of how you think about yourself, both positive and negative. You will begin to identify and locate feelings in your soul and in your body. You will lose your fear of having feelings. And most wondrously, as you move through your days you will find your affirmations appearing in your thoughts spontaneously, replacing a negative thought you usually would have experienced. For example, perhaps your boss gives you some feedback on your work. You may find yourself smiling and thinking, *I, Pat am intelligent,* instead of the usual tightening of your gut and the old *I, Pat am stupid.* In other words, the healing power of our own minds and bodies creates the final transformation of our hurt into strength. All we have to do is the repetition of our affirmations.

There are many effective methods for the healing process of repetition.

written affirmations

Written affirmations are valuable because the act of writing something down means you are using both body and mind. This is more powerful than just thinking nice thoughts about yourself. The other advantage of written affirmations is that they allow you to make a record of the negative belief systems you continue to hold, but are possibly unaware of. This information lets you know how important your affirmations are and how important it is for you to continue the healing repetition process. A written record of positive thoughts or beliefs you hold about yourself will also emerge. Gradually, as you continue the healing process of repetition, the positive beliefs will overcome the negative beliefs until the negative belief system will feel like an echo from some distant past in another life.

> **TIP**
>
> Remember an important principal of self-affirmation work, *Love brings up everything like itself for the purpose of healing.* This means that negative thoughts are coming up for the purpose of healing.

Written affirmations should include all three voices. That is, *I, you,* and *she.* This will allow you discover any negativity in all the relationships in your life and heal it. Written affirmations should also include a response column which will allow you to write down your response to each affirmation as you repeat it over and over. You may type, key in on a computer, or handwrite your affirmations. All use the body and the mind.

I recommend that you do at least one page of written affirmations per day with each voice using about one-third of the page. It is good to do your self-affirmation work in the morning before your day starts or in the evening before sleeping. Once your self-affirmation work is done for the day, put it away and forget about it. Your work is done for the day. Your body and mind will do the rest. You will find the affirmations spontaneously appearing in your thoughts. This always feels good to me, and it should feel good to you too. You may have a set of affirmations to complete. Use a separate page for each affirmation.

An example of the process is followed by a blank form or chart which you may use in the workbook, but a more valuable use would be to use the form for copying, keeping this workbook form as your original.

A WRITTEN AFFIRMATION PROCESS SAMPLE

Voice	Name	Affirmation	Response
I	Pat	am intelligent.	I don't believe that.
I	Pat	am intelligent.	Oh sure!
I	Pat	am intelligent.	How come I can't spell?
I	Pat	am intelligent.	Well, I've read lots of books.
I	Pat	am intelligent.	How did I get here?
I	Pat	am intelligent.	I did get through that class.
I	Pat	am intelligent.	Maybe I should sign up for school full time.
You	Pat	are intelligent.	You're really dumb!
You	Pat	are intelligent.	Born in a barn?
You	Pat	are intelligent.	Stomach hurts.
You	Pat	are intelligent.	Can't think at all.
You	Pat	are intelligent.	Wait a minute, I'm not so stupid.
You	Pat	are intelligent.	My math teacher said I'm smart.
You	Pat	are intelligent.	I did get an A.
She	Pat	is intelligent.	Numb. Checked out.
She	Pat	is intelligent.	Nothing in my head at all.
She	Pat	is intelligent.	Do people know about me?
She	Pat	is intelligent.	I'm afraid of school.
She	Pat	is intelligent.	Dogs like me.
She	Pat	is intelligent.	Mrs. Jones said she knew I could do math.
She	Pat	is intelligent.	Nothing again. I can't feel my hands.

TIP

The responses in the Response Column don't have to be logical or even make sense. They are valid because they are your responses. You may not understand some of your responses immediately or even be surprised by them.

TIP

Except for changing the voice and the appropriate verbs to match, the affirmation *stays exactly the same.* You will not get the best results if you change your wording and do not keep it precise. The part of our brain which hangs onto both negative and positive thoughts likes these thoughts to be simple and exactly the same.

TIP

Put your written self-affirmation work in a safe place. You have a right to privacy in your self-affirmation work. By keeping your work safe, you are showing yourself respect.

A WRITTEN AFFIRMATION PROCESS

Voice	Name	Affirmation	Response

I _____

_____

_____

_____

_____

You _____

_____

_____

_____

_____

She _____

_____

_____

_____

_____

TIP

Keep this form for copying so that you have ready-made affirmation sheets for your use.

recorded affirmations

For those of you who prefer speaking to writing, the use of a tape recorder to record spoken affirmations is also a powerful method of the healing repetition process. It may be helpful to have the affirmation written out in the three voices so that you get the most complete affirmation process. The technique is to speak the affirmation into the recorder a specified number of times (determined by you – maybe you think seven is your lucky number). Make certain to use each voice (I, you, and she) in your spoken process. Then rewind the tape and listen to your own voice speaking the affirmations.

This method has all the necessary ingredients. There is the mind/body connection. With written or keyboard listings of the affirmations, both the mind and the hands participate. With the recording method, both the mind and voice participate. What is not present is the response column. I do not recommend interrupting the rhythm of spoken affirmations by stopping to record the response to each affirmation. The power of the spoken affirmation is diminished somehow by interrupting the rhythm. The method, however, is highly effective. If you feel a need to record your responses, you could make verbal notes on the tape at the end of your session, or take notes of your responses in a journal kept for this purpose. You may wish to keep your recorded tapes, but many people use the same tape over and over. Either method is correct.

spoken affirmations: with yourself, with a partner

If you spend a great deal of time alone in your car (e.g., commuting to and from work, driving to appointments, or driving your child or children here and there) the spoken affirmation process may be ideal for you. Basically, the process is exactly the same as the *Recorded Affirmation* process outlined above. There is just no tape to listen to when you are finished with your self-affirmation session. The key to the affirmation process is always the same; exact repetition of the affirmations is the basis of the healing of verbal-emotional abuse.

Spoken affirmations with a partner offer a way to share your affirmation work with others, and also to support others in their affirmation work. This may be of vital importance if you are a survivor with children. Children usually have fun with the affirmation process. One very helpful affirmation with children, who are now out of the abusive situation, but whose sense of safety is still shaky, is *You are safe now.* Children need to hear this from their mothers and other adults, and they need to know that their mothers are safe now as well.

The partner affirmations work like this. The partners sit comfortably facing each other, if possible. The partners decide on the number of repetitions they are going to use in their work of healing repetition. One person in the partnership starts with, *I, Patty, am safe now.* (As in all self-affirmation work, it is important to use your name. With partnership affirmations, the use of the partner's name is also part of the work.) The partner responds by saying, *That's right.* After the agreed upon number of repetitions has been completed, the supporting partner then starts the affirmation process with *You, Patty, are safe now.* Patty then responds with *That's right.* Partners then switch so that both partners get to experience the affirmations in both the *I* and *you* voices.

TIP

An easy way to keep count of the number of repetitions is to use your fingers. If this seems child-like to you, good. Self-affirmation work is essentially about discovering and healing the wise child within.

TIP

The physical presence of a partner in your self-affirmation work will make visible your physical responses to the affirmations. You may end up laughing, crying, stop breathing, or flush in embarrassment. The solution is to use the slow easy breathing described in *Getting Started: A Meditation.* If your partner is having similar trouble, support your partner by conscious breathing, or say *breathe.* Then breathe with your partner while resuming the healing process of repetition.

TIP

Courtesy in partnership affirmation work includes asking your partner if she or he has an affirmation to work on in that session. Partners do not have to have the same affirmations in order to work with each other.

A PARTNERSHIP AFFIRMATION PROCESS WITH
PATTY AND HER MOTHER, RENE

Patty	*I, Patty am safe now.*	Rene	*That's right.*
Patty	*I, Patty am safe now.*	Rene	*That's right.*
Patty	*I, Patty am safe now.*	Rene	*That's right.*
Patty	*I, Patty am safe now.*	Rene	*That's right.*
Patty	*I, Patty am safe now.*	Rene	*That's right.*
Patty	*I, Patty am safe now.*	Rene	*That's right.*
Patty	*I, Patty am safe now.*	Rene	*That's right*

Rene	*You, Patty are safe now.*	Patty	*That's right.*
Rene	*You, Patty are safe now.*	Patty	*That's right.*
Rene	*You, Patty are safe now.*	Patty	*That's right.*
Rene	*You, Patty are safe now.*	Patty	*That's right.*
Rene	*You, Patty are safe now.*	Patty	*That's right.*
Rene	*You, Patty are safe now.*	Patty	*That's right.*
Rene.	*You, Patty are safe now.*	Patty	*That's right.*

Rene	*I, Rene am safe now.*	Patty	*That's right.*
Rene	*I, Rene am safe now.*	Patty	*That's right.*
Rene	*I, Rene am safe now.*	Patty	*That's right.*
Rene	*I, Rene am safe now.*	Patty	*That's right.*
Rene	*I, Rene am safe now.*	Patty	*That's right.*
Rene	*I, Rene am safe now.*	Patty	*That's right.*
Rene	*I, Rene am safe now.*	Patty	*That's right.*

Patty	*You, Rene are safe now.*	Rene	*That's right.*
Patty	*You, Rene are safe now.*	Rene	*That's right.*
Patty	*You, Rene are safe now.*	Rene	*That's right.*
Patty	*You, Rene are safe now.*	Rene	*That's right.*
Patty	*You, Rene are safe now.*	Rene	*That's right.*
Patty	*You, Rene are safe now.*	Rene	*That's right.*
Patty	*You, Rene are safe now.*	Rene	*That's right.*

Self-affirmation work is one effective method for overcoming verbal-emotional abuse. It is a self-empowerment experience based on the identification of core negative beliefs which have been created by verbal-emotional abuse, the transformation of these core negative beliefs into affirmations, and the repetition of these affirmations in order to facilitate the healing process.

The overcoming of verbal-emotional abuse is a key element in career and life planning because the nature of career and life planning is to challenge any negative thought systems, including beliefs about your competence in the worlds of parenting, waged work and education, and your right to make a life meaningful to you.

Now that you have gathered your words of power or your tools, you are ready for the next steps. That is, claiming your heritage as a working woman in Western Civilization by *moving through the flower*.

section II: the process – moving through the flower

Moving through the flower is a process that is available to all of us, a process that can lead to a place where we can express our humanity and values as women through our work and in our lives and in so doing, perhaps we can also reach across the great gulf between masculine and feminine and gently, tenderly, but firmly heal it.

Chicago, 1977, p. 206

introduction

Through the Flower is both the title of one of Judy Chicago's books and one of her paintings, a luminous work I saw hanging in the National Museum of Women in the Arts in Washington, DC in 1991. It is a painting which beckons and shimmers with invitation. The invitation is to step through, into another reality, a woman's reality. The purpose of this section is to extend this invitation to you as well.

The sensual and magnificent visual and written expression of this reality has been created by the artist Judy Chicago in collaboration with hundreds of women and men, in a series of art projects starting with *Womanhouse* (1971), then *The Dinner Party* (1979), and *The Birth Project* (1985). In each of these efforts, Chicago has guided both women and men in going *through the flower* by exploring the meanings of women's work on many levels simultaneously. Her latest eight-year effort was completed in a partnership with her husband, Donald Woodman. *The Holocaust Project* (1993) also explores women's work within the human tragedy we know as the Holocaust.

Chicago's books offer rich descriptions of the complexities of women's work. There is her journal process which describes her struggle as a woman artist, writer, and teacher. Her observations on the damaged work lives and work habits of women are, perhaps, the most important commentary now available on the work psychology of women. Then there is the writing of those who have shared the collaborative art-making process with Chicago. Both women and men write about their experience of Chicago as a role model, teacher, and an inspiring and challenging guide. Photographs in all of the books document not only the artwork, but also the process of creating the art. The content of the writing and of the visual expressions (photographs of the art work, the art making process, the graphic design of the books themselves) are also explorations of women's work. The books are *Through the Flower: My Struggle As A Woman Artist* (1977), *The Dinner Party: A Symbol of Our Heritage* (1979), *Embroidering Our Heritage: The Dinner Party Needlework* (1980), and *The Holocaust Project: From Darkness Into Light* (1993).

RESOURCE – Through the Flower, Inc. is a nonprofit organization which owns and controls the showing of *The Dinner Party*. The effort to house *The Dinner Party* in its own museum in Santa Fe, New Mexico is also part of this organization's responsibility. To join Through the Flower as a member, to host dinner parties for *The Dinner Party, to* make contributions toward the values expressed in *The*

Dinner Party, or to obtain more information regarding the work of Judy Chicago; write P.O. Box 8138, Santa Fe, NM 87504.

And then there is the glory of the artwork. Both *The Dinner Party* and *The Birth Project* raise women's traditional needlework to the level of high art. *The Dinner Party* is a celebration of women's china painting traditions. Both the needlework and the china painting are used to make visible a woman's reality, whether that reality is within the world of achievement as a scientist, mystic, freedom fighter, or goddess (*The Dinner Party*), or within the world of a woman's body (*The Birth Project*). Chicago's art explores both the sacred and the mundane aspects of women's realities. She makes visible the mundane, tedious aspects of women's invisible unwaged work, and she celebrates the erased and obliterated achievements of the women we have lost.

One example is Theodora. She is, or should be, a hero to every abuse survivor. She started life as an actor, and became the Empress of Byzantium. "She issued an imperial decree making it illegal—and punishable by death—to entice a woman into prostitution, and she turned one of her palaces into an institution where prostitutes could go to start new lives" (Chicago, 1979). Theodora also instituted the death penalty for rape, and passed laws against the mistreatment of women by their husbands. She lived long before our so-called liberated era, from 508 to 548 AD.

> **TIP**
>
> *The Dinner Party: A Symbol of Our Heritage* is an excellent resource for finding a guide to call upon in the guided meditation suggested in *Overcoming Verbal-Emotional Abuse.*

What is missing from Chicago's contributions to our developing theories of women's work is the realities of poor women of every ethnic group and color. The hundreds of volunteers who collaborated with Chicago over the years were generally drawn from the educated middle class, usually white. Who else has the luxury of taking months or years away from the business of making a living? And Chicago herself writes, "As I worked on the research for *The Dinner Party* and then on the piece itself, a nagging voice kept reminding me that the women whose plates I was painting, whose runners we were embroidering, whose names we were firing onto the porcelain floor, were primarily women of the ruling classes. History has been written from the point of view of those who have been in power. It is not an objective record of the human race—we do not know the history of humankind. A true history would allow us to see the mingled efforts of peoples of all colors and sexes, all countries and races, all seeing the universe in their own diverse ways."

Therefore when you do not see your brown face, your ivory skin, your black eyes reflected back at you as you pour over the photographs of women at work in Chicago's books, I refer you to *Making Face, Making Soul: Haciendo Caras* (1990) edited by Gloria Anzaldua; *Spider Woman's Granddaughters* (1989) edited by Paula Gunn Allen; *Getting Home Alive* (1986) by Aurora Levins Morales and Rosario Morales; *Wild Swans: Three Daughters of China* (1991) by Jung Chang; *Women's*

Work: The Art of Pablita Velarde (1993) by Sally Hyer; *Lakota Woman* (1990) by Mary Crow Dog; *The Alchemy of Race and Rights: The Diary of a Law Professor* (1991) by Patricia J. Williams; *If I Had a Hammer: Women's Work in Poetry, Fiction, and Photographs* (1990) edited by Sandra Martz; *Women in the Global Factory* (1989) by Annette Feuntes and Barbara Ehrenreich; and even the *Occupational Outlook Handbook, 1992 – 1993 Edition* developed by the U.S. Department of Labor Bureau of Labor Statistics. And finally I refer you to the famous and profound words from Zora Neale Hurston's book, *Their Eyes Were Watching God* (1937), "De nigger woman is de mule uh de world so fur as Ah can see."

Chicago's efforts are finally only a beginning. *The Dinner Party* research took place in the 70s, and helped to lay the groundwork for women's studies as we know it today. You will notice that the list above consists of books published within the past five years (except for Hurston who has just been rediscovered). These books are also just the beginning of what women of color have to tell us all.

What I suggest is that the movement *through the flower* is unique for each woman because it is based in *her* reality, whatever that might be. Chicago's work does not offer the only passage, but it is the most explicit and richly articulated passage I have found. It is my hope that the Workbook is inclusive enough so that each of you can discover what it is you need to do to go *through the flower*.

Chicago's contributions to our thinking about women's work are as follows: first, women's work, whether is be that of queen or mule, needs to be made visible. Second, women's work is worthy of analysis, respect, and celebration. Third, women often have a problematic, damaged relationship to their own work and work lives. Fourth, women can heal this damage by moving *through the flower*, into their own reality.

The first chapter in this section, *Making Your Work Visible*, addresses not only the importance of your personal history, but your relationship to women's history as part of a continuity of women's achievements over time. The second chapter, *Analyzing, Respecting and Celebrating Your Work*, is a process which allows your to take an inventory of your current skill development. The third chapter, *Understanding Your Vocational Impairment*, summarizes all that has gone before, and helps you to make the next leap forward. This chapter prepares you for the last section of the Workbook, *The Plan – Re-Weaving Your Own Life and Work*.

seven

---

making your work visible

I thought the images on the plates would convey the fact that the women I planned to represent had been swallowed up and obscured by history instead of being recognized and honored.

Judy Chicago, 1979, p. 8

If you think that the making of your work, or any woman's work, visible is a simple minded task, consider the fact that *The Dinner Party,* which has been exhibited 14 times in six countries and seen by almost a million viewers is now in storage and is without permanent housing. The suppression of *The Dinner Party* is an expression of the current global economic system which is based on the suppression of women's work (Waring, 1988). Chicago's nonprofit organization, Through the Flower, has now taken on the task of raising money to house *The Dinner Party.* You, too, will need to take on the task of building your own record and your own housing for your achievements.

The historian, Gerda Lerner, points out that women have a different relationship to history than men. Men benefit from the achievements of the men who have gone before them. They stand on the shoulders of other men. They preserve their histories by creating institutions which sustain the values they wish to keep. Women, by contrast, are doomed to reinvent the wheel over and over. This is why *The Dinner Party*, a symbolic history of women's achievements in Western Civilization, is so important. This is why your record of your own achievements is so important. Without your own record, how can you link yourself to the women who have gone before you without feeling overwhelmed and intimidated? And how can you examine the reality of your achievements without a framework, a context in which to understand your position as a woman? Without this framework, we are doomed to see ourselves as imperfect and inadequate men. And if we do not possess our own personal histories, how can we become actors in the making of women's history? If we cannot make our own work visible, then we will lose *The Dinner Party* and our daughters and granddaughters will have to reinvent the wheel over and over again. The process of making visible your own achievements is not only part of your recovery, but also a way of linking to the achievements of the women who have gone before and the women who will come after you are gone.

You may choose the order in which you wish to complete this work, but if you are like most abuse survivors, you may leave out your most important achievement, the saving of your own life. Or perhaps, it might be the saving of the lives of your child or children.

saving my own life

From my studies of women's art and literature and my research into women's lives — undertaken as a part of my search for my own tradition as a woman and an artist — I had concluded that the general lack of knowledge of our heritage as women was pivotal in our continued oppression as women. Because we were educated to think that women had never achieved anything of significance, it was easy to believe that we were incapable of accomplishing important work.
Judy Chicago, 1980, p. 8

The story of how you saved your own life or the life of your child or your children is a story which deserves to be recorded. This record could take the form of drawings, or writing, or speaking on video or audiotape. This story probably has no ending because as we go through the life-long process of recovery, we understand more and more about how we saved our own lives, how we survived, what our survival means, who we were then, and who we are now. Therefore, we may start out the making of the story of ourselves as hero with one sentence or even one word. That's okay. More will come as you move through your recovery. Others may find that the story rushes out of you like water caught behind an old logjam. Record as much as you can in many ways as you can. You may choose to tinker with the record later, making it clearer as you become clearer. The point is to begin.

TIP

See the guided meditation in the chapter, *Overcoming Verbal-Emotional Abuse,* if you feel a need for protection in doing this work. Lighting a candle or burning incense or sweet grass can also create that sacred space in which your work becomes possible. Using colored pencils to draw boundary lines around the pages in your journal or in this workbook, and then writing or drawing your story inside of that is another method of making your story sacred and yourself safe.

TIP

The journal paradox (whether or not your journal is a written record or an audio or video tape record) is that while the journal is meant to be private, it is also meant to be shared. *However, this* sharing is to be done when you want, with whom you want, and which portions you see fit to give. (e.g., You may feel that your children are too young or too fragile right now to understand how you saved their lives, and your own, but you may wish to share it with them later).

RESOURCE – *The Courage to Heal Workbook* (1990) by Laura Davis offers the healing exercises of *freewriting* and *making collages.* Natalie Goldberg's *Wild Mind: Living the Writer's Life* (1990) is another excellent guide to releasing your writing muscles.

TIP

   Fill in as much detail as you can. Add detail later as you remember it (e.g., I saved money for weeks so I could pay the fare for myself and the kids for a taxicab. I packed my favorite clothes and kept them at a friend's house. It took ten tries, but I finally made it. I made a complete escape plan for my self which included....).

I am the hero of my own life. This is the story of how I save myself (my child, my children). (e.g., I reported my husband to the police, and they arrested him. I took myself and my children to a safe house. I ran away from home and lived on the streets. I left my body when I was molested. I played dead when the rapist attacked me. I reported my harasser to an attorney, and we filed a lawsuit. I punched my battering pimp in the jaw, and contacted the Council for Prostitution Alternatives. I asked for help.)

_____

_____

_____

_____

_____

_____

_____

_____

_____

assembling the records of my achievements

Slowly the files grew. Cataloging the material alphabetically and by country, century, and profession, we began to assemble the fractured pieces of our heritage which would eventually appear on the 2,300 twelve-inch, triangular porcelain tiles that make up the Heritage Floor.

Judy Chicago, 1979, p. 19

Another step in this process of making your work visible is to explore your own library, your archives for the documents of your own life. These archives could be the trunk in your mother's basement where your report cards, high school album, and baby pictures are kept. If these treasures had to be abandoned in the saving of your own life, do your best to recreate them by making lists of what these treasures were. You may also choose to obtain old family photographs from other family members, or write to your grade school, high school, trade school, business college, or university to get your records. You may have lost journals or school books with your notes in them because your abuser forced you to burn them. You have a right to either attempt to recreate them or, at least, make a memorial for them, even if it is just a note in your new journal, or an altar in honor of your lost history. Records may include diplomas, certificates, transcripts, calendars, diaries, letters, birth certificates, medical records (including emergency room records), paintings, drawings, or other artwork you have done including needlework; and your child's (children's) records including baby books, report cards, birth certificates, and photographs.

Records from your waged work life should also be gathered. This is important for everyone, but is particularly crucial for sexual harassment survivors whose perceptions of their work lives are frequently distorted by the harasser(s) (e.g., You got the best performance evaluation ever, but then got fired). These records can include check stubs, performance evaluations, company newsletters, memos you have written, an example of work you've done (if possible), photographs of yourself and fellow workers, job descriptions.

It is also important to gather documents which might be crucial to your own ethnic and racial history. For example, Patricia J. Williams' examination of the contract of sale of her great-great-grandmother immediately leads to a piercing of the veil around the lives of African-American women in this country. Williams (1991, pp. 17-19) writes, "This story is what inspired my interest in the interplay of notions of public and private, of family and market; of male and female, of molestation and the law." In other words, her discovery of this contract changed her, and her work life as a law professor. A discovery like Williams' is unlikely to occur in your first assembling of records. However, it is legitimate to consider such documents as part of your story. Your story is connected to the stories of all women, but most closely to the women who share your ethnic, racial, cultural, and religious heritage.

Now that you have this stack of stuff in a pile in front of you, what do you do with it? Make lists, of course. Six lists should do it, but if you find you need more categories, feel free to make more lists. Arranging your documents, photographs, and other artifacts according to these categories will help you to make the lists more efficiently. The categories are **Childhood Achievements: Education and Work; Adult Educational Achievements; Adult Unwaged Work Achievements; Adult Waged Work Achievements; Women Who Have Come Before Me;** and **Miscellaneous.**

TIP

    This is a process which may be best done with a friend, your recovery group, your therapist, or rehabilitation counselor. It is a process which may take days, weeks, or months (e.g., I travelled to the Chicago area with my friend, the poet Jeanne Simonoff, where we looked for the traces of her mother's life which had been erased by her own family. When Jeanne was three years old, her mother died, leaving Jeanne without her mother's heritage. We found Jeanne's mother's college records at Northwestern University. This process may be particularly important for you if you were adopted, or have lost your parents in some way).

Childhood Achievements: Education and Work (e.g., You may wish to list the highest grade level completed, the best grades you received, the scores for attendance or social skills. Don't forget the unwaged work you did as a child. Girl children are frequently expected to provide complete childcare and housework services at a very early age. Looking at old photographs of yourself in relation to younger children can trigger memories of such work. List any hobbies, crafts, athletic or artistic skills you developed as a child. List work for which you were paid. If you can remember how much you were paid, write that down too.)

Date   Your Age   Achievement

_____

_____

_____

_____

_____

_____

_____

_____

_____

_____

_____

_____

_____

_____

Date   Your Age   Achievement

_____

_____

_____

_____

_____

_____

_____

_____

_____

_____

_____

_____

_____

_____

_____

_____

_____

_____

Adult Educational Achievements (e.g., List all completed educational efforts since high school. If you did not graduate from high school, but have taken classes, completed your GED, read the newspaper everyday, read lots of books, list those accomplishments. List degrees and certificates. List all the times you started school, but had to drop out to appease your abuser. List the classes you took while you were enduring abuse, and passed anyway. List the classes you are taking now. List the therapy and recovery work you've done. List all the times you got up the courage to even go onto a college campus. Called to sign up for the GED test.)

Date   Your Age   Achievement

_____

_____

_____

_____

_____

_____

_____

_____

_____

_____

_____

_____

_____

Date   Your Age   Achievement

_____

_____

_____

_____

_____

_____

_____

_____

_____

_____

_____

_____

_____

_____

_____

_____

_____

_____

_____

Adult Unwaged Work Achievements (e.g., List your parenting accomplishments such as creating clean, clothed, well-fed, strong children and happy children. List the learning you have done to become a better parent such as your parenting classes, recovery work at the battered women's center, going to parent and teacher meetings at your child's school. Include your own parenting of yourself on this list such as making sure that you get proper rest, food, clothing, shelter, and structure. List all the housework, gardening, cooking, driving, and grocery shopping work you do. You may want to carry a notebook around with you for a few days and jot these tasks down as you go. If you receive welfare income, you may want to list what it takes to keep those checks coming in, and what you have to do to live on a welfare check. List what you had to do to get to the emergency room after being raped and/or beaten. List the work of surviving the emergency room procedures.)

Date   Your Age   Achievement

_____

_____

_____

_____

_____

_____

_____

_____

_____

_____

_____

_____

Date   Your Age   Achievement

_____

_____

_____

_____

_____

_____

_____

_____

_____

_____

_____

_____

_____

_____

_____

_____

_____

_____

_____

_____

Adult Waged Work Achievements (e.g., List all the jobs you have held in chronological order. List the wages you received, the length of time on the job, and a brief description of the job duties. List any promotions, awards, or raises you received. List the jobs you kept even though you were being abused at the time. List the jobs you lost because of traumatic abuse. List your self-employment endeavors, including child care in your home for others. List the work you did in your husband's business, if you received wages for it. If not, list this work under **Unwaged Work** above.)

Date   Your Age   Achievement

_____

_____

_____

_____

_____

_____

_____

_____

_____

_____

_____

_____

_____

_____

Date   Your Age   Achievement

_____

_____

_____

_____

_____

_____

_____

_____

_____

_____

_____

_____

_____

_____

_____

_____

_____

_____

_____

_____

Women Who Have Come Before Me (e.g., Patricia William's discovery of her great-great grandmother's contract of sale, or Jeanne Simonoff's location of her mother's college records. Have you discovered some records of the women of your own family, or from your own ethnic or religious heritage? Perhaps a mythical or religious figure such as the Blessed Virgin Mary has been an inspiration to you as you've moved through your waged and unwaged work life. Perhaps a teacher or a boss has changed your thoughts about your work and yourself as a worker. List the names of such women. How do you feel about them? About their work? What is it about their work that influences your work? Describe your connection to them through your work.)

Date   Your Age   Achievement

_____

_____

_____

_____

_____

_____

_____

_____

_____

_____

_____

_____

_____

_____

Date   Your Age   Achievement

_____

_____

_____

_____

_____

_____

_____

_____

_____

_____

_____

_____

_____

_____

_____

_____

_____

Miscellaneous (e.g., This section might be useful for listing achievements resulting from artistic activities, hobbies, sports or volunteer work. Independent study into your own ethnic and cultural background as a woman could be listed here. Maybe you designed your dream house or took a trip to Mexico on your own. List such accomplishments here if they haven't fit elsewhere. Make a list of all the poems you've written, the art pieces you've created, the songs you've sung, the recovery work you've completed.)

Date   Your Age   Achievement

_____

_____

_____

_____

_____

_____

_____

_____

_____

_____

_____

_____

_____

_____

Date   Your Age   Achievement

_____

_____

_____

_____

_____

_____

_____

_____

_____

_____

_____

_____

_____

_____

_____

_____

_____

_____

You have just made yourself visible as a worker. The claiming of your identity as a worker is a revolutionary act.

You have just created a document which can be used by you in developing a vocational plan, in discussing your work goals with your rehabilitation counselor, your attorney, in applying for a job, in writing a new resume.

You have just taken your place in the history of women's achievements.

eight

---

analyzing, respecting, and celebrating your work

With no research skills and little scholarly background, team members plundered the libraries for books about women. They learned to cut through the biases of history which usually described, not the woman's achievements, but her physical attributes and the men in her life. The research team gradually developed its skills... I watched them all undergo a process very similar to my own: As they learned about their history as women, their sense of themselves changed. Their initial lack of confidence was replaced by an understanding of their historic circumstances and a determination to share the information they were finding with other women.

Judy Chicago, 1979

Learning "to cut through the biases of history" is never more important than when thinking about the work of women since the work women do is devalued because they do it. This means that women receive less pay, less status, and less recognition for their work. Child care is the supreme example of this point, although any waged occupation where women are found in large numbers generally has less status and less pay than comparable work done by men. The devaluing of the work of women by patriarchal culture has its most direct expression in sexual harassment. This method of degrading a woman's identity as a worker is a way of letting all women know that no matter what your work is and how well you do it, because you are a woman, your work will never be as good as a man's.

The purpose of this chapter is to give you a defense against such slander. The method is the transferable skills analysis of your waged and unwaged work history based on *The Dictionary of Occupational Titles' Definitions of Worker Functions* (1991, pp. 1005-1007). The advantage of a transferable skills analysis is that it undercuts the stereotypes about women's work by redefining the work in terms of skills rather than by job titles which tend to be based on gender. This, in turn, will give you a new way of thinking and talking about your own work history, as well as opening the way for you to see how to develop a new and more satisfying work life for yourself. The other advantage in this method is that if you are working with a vocational expert in the preparation of a lawsuit, or with a rehabilitation counselor in a rehabilitation system, you will have handed your expert or your counselor a valuable tool to use on your behalf. This is because a transferable skills analysis is one of the tools of the rehabilitation professions.

RESOURCE – Richard Nelson Bolles' *1992 What Color Is Your Parachute?* from Ten Speed Press contains a very complete and well known transferable skills analysis method which you might wish to investigate. This analysis is also available as a booklet titled, *The Quick Job Hunting Map.*

The Dictionary of Occupational Titles (1991, p. 1005) "is based on the premise that every job requires a worker to function, to some degree, in relation to Data, People, and Things." The relationships or activities in which workers engage are listed below.

DATA	PEOPLE	THINGS
0 Synthesizing	0 Mentoring	0 Setting Up
1 Coordinating	1 Negotiating	1 Precision Working
2 Analyzing	2 Instructing	2 Operating-Controlling
3 Compiling	3 Supervising	3 Driving-Operating
4 Computing	4 Diverting	4 Manipulating
5 Copying	5 Persuading	5 Tending
6 Comparing	6 Speaking – Signaling	6 Feeding-Offbearing
	7 Serving	7 Handling
	8 Taking Instructions-Helping	

The numbers listed before each activity are part of a numeric code in *The Dictionary of Occupational Titles.* These numbers also refer to the level of complexity required to perform the activity. The higher the number, the lower the skill level required. This listing also assumes that if you can perform the highest level function, you can also perform all the other functions below it. So if you can mentor your children, you are also able to negotiate, or serve, or help someone else. It doesn't work the other way, however. That is, you may be able to copy some data, but not be able to analyze it or make sense out of it at your present level of skill development.

The career of Judy Chicago provides us with a way to illustrate the Data, People, and Things model. The achievements of this artist encompass every aspect of the functions listed within the model. This extraordinary woman has not only created art with her own hands (Things), she has written about the process in her many books (Data), and she has done this work in collaboration with hundreds of people over the years as a mentor, leader, and visionary (People). Most of us are not so gifted, nor are we so committed to furthering the development of our skills.

Chicago's statements about the development of her skills and knowledge base are breathtaking in their audacity, and a challenge to us all to not let mere ignorance stop us from what we want to accomplish. She writes, "After I finished college, I decided to go to auto body school and learn to spray paint, something several male artists had discussed doing. I was the only woman among 250 men....I learned quite a bit that was actually beneficial to me as an artist, the most important being an understanding of the role of craft" (1979, p. 37). Other ventures into craft included plastics, fireworks, and china painting (Chicago, 1980, p. 10). *The Dinner Party* (1979) has a research base of more than one thousand books, and *The Holocaust Project* (1993) alone has involved more than eight years of research. But despite these achievements, Chicago has had to face a hard truth, "Now it is clear to me that to expect men to validate one for challenging male dominance (which is what a woman artist implicitly does, simply by being a woman and artist) is entirely fantastic" (1979, p. 43).

Therefore, if you have the expectation that the development of your skills and knowledge base will meet with male approval, you may be in for a shock. If you are a survivor of sexual harassment on the job or in the classroom, understand that the purpose of this harassment was to keep you from developing your skills and knowledge base and/or to keep you from using your skills and knowledge. If you are a rape survivor, chances are your rape trauma occurred during the statistically vulnerable years for rape (between the ages of 13 and 26) (Russell, 1984, pp. 80-81). These are also the years when most women develop the skills and knowledge base they will use for the rest of their lives. It is my contention that marital rape, acquaintance rape, stranger rape, and institutionalized rape (prostitution) function to prevent women and girls from gaining the skills and knowledge they need to reach their maximum potential, to prevent women and girls from taking their power, to assert their rights to a living wage, a quality work life. It matters little whether the overwhelmingly male perpetrators of these crimes are consciously aware of this effect. No conspiracy theory is necessary. Women and girls give up their vocational aspirations every time a woman is abused.

And as we learned in the *Introduction,* woman battering has been conceptualized as a form of slavery by the legal theorist Joyce E. McConnell. This analysis means that even if a woman develops a sophisticated skills and knowledge base, it does not belong to her. She is a slave. Her work is to be used as her master sees fit. The fruits of her labor are also not her own. She may be forced to sign away her house, her bank account in order to live.

In all of these situations, a woman's vocational development becomes contaminated. Some women lose the link between their productive activity and money. Some women can go to school, but cannot function in the workplace. Other women cannot imagine being without a man to support them. Some women lose entire occupations or professions because of the trauma which results from the abuse. These women are forced to find other occupations to earn a living. Such women are vulnerable to being underemployed. That is, working in jobs which are far below their educational attainment level. Some women become disabled and join the ranks of the unemployed. Statistically, disabled women who have work earn less than $10,000 per year (McNeil, 1983). Disabled women who are traumatized by abuse may give up their unceasing struggle for dignity and independence after the abuse experience. In short, damage to your transferable skills and knowledge base is damage to your earning capacity.

The development of your skills and knowledge base does not take place in a vacuum. Your best chance for using your skills and knowledge occurs when other women are either working in your field of endeavor or have at least established a female presence. Even such a gifted and determined woman as Judy Chicago was prevented from being certified as a pyrotechnician because of sexual harassment. She was impeded in her artmaking because without certification she could not shoot her own fireworks shows. She did not use pyrotechniques in her artmaking again until she met a woman who had succeeded in becoming certified (1979, p. 58-59). The point is that as a woman worker your work takes place within the context of the history of women's work whether you like it or not. Never underestimate the power of knowing that another woman has gone before you. Your understanding of the history of women is the foundation upon which your skills and knowledge base needs to rest.

a transferable skills analysis of my achievement history

The work you completed in the previous chapter will now be harvested for the kernels of your current skills and knowledge. You may be pleasantly surprised at the number of skills you possess. Most people underestimate their skill levels.

In this chapter, you will examine each of the exercises completed in the previous chapter, starting with *Saving My Own Life,* and ending with *Miscellaneous.* As you perform your examination, you will identify the skills you used to save your own life, or care for your child (unwaged work), or perform your job (waged work). This analysis will be based on the Data, People, and Things model as outlined above. The *Data, People, and Things Charts* are set up in pairs. One chart has been completed by me so that you will have an example to refer to when you complete your transferable skills analysis on your skills chart.

> **TIP**
>
> Your skills and knowledge base can be developed and enhanced at any age, but first it is important to understand what your skills are now. Then it becomes possible to design the best plan for developing your skills and knowledge so that *your* needs and interests are satisfied.

TIP

Since most of us survivors either are, or have been, members of the If-I-Can-Do-It-It-Must-Not-Be- Much-Club, you may find yourself swamped by waves of criticism or self-hatred while doing the analysis. This is a signal to go back to the chapter, *Overcoming Verbal-Emotional Abuse.* You may wish to create an affirmation to use before and after working on your transferable skills analysis (e.g., I, Patty, am intelligent and capable).

TIP

It may seem puzzling to analyze the skills of *The Women Who Have Come Before Me* as part of *your* transferable skills analysis, but the skills we admire in others are usually skills we would like to have for ourselves. Therefore when you complete this part of the analysis, you will have created a list of dreams and goals for yourself. As we have learned in the chapter, *Naming the Trauma,* symptoms of post-traumatic stress disorder or of complex post-traumatic stress disorder include damage to the creative process and a sense of hopelessness about the future. This part of the transferable skills analysis is designed to help you get around, under, over, or through such damage.

TIP

You may not have used all of the worker functions listed on the *Data, People, Things Charts.* Most of us are not skilled at everything. For example, you may not know how to drive a car. If so, you will probably not be completing the *Driving-Operating* section under Things. That's okay. In these exercises, what you do not complete will be just as important as what you do complete, but that discussion is reserved for the next chapter.

SAMPLE DATA SKILLS CHART

DATA: Information, knowledge, and conceptions, related to data, people, or things, obtained by observation, investigation, interpretation, visualization, and mental creation. Data are intangible and include numbers, words, symbols, ideas, concepts, and oral verbalization.

My Achievement History	1. Saving My Own Life	2. Childhood Achievements	3. Adult Educational Achievements
Synthesizing: Integrating analyses of data to discover facts and/or develop knowledge concepts or interpretation.	*I completed therapy.*	*I wrote poetry.*	*I completed my senior thesis.*
Coordinating: Determining time, place, and sequence of operations or actions to be taken on the basis of analyzing data; executing determinations and/or reporting on events.	*I organized the escape.*	*I organized the kids for snow play.*	*I organized my class outing.*
Analyzing: Examining and evaluating data Presenting alternative actions in relation to the evaluation is frequently involved.	*I read the materials on abuse.*	*I figured out that I could make more money.*	*I figured out how to take classes, work, and parent.*
Compiling: Gathering, collating, or classifying information about data, people, or things. Reporting and/or carrying out a prescribed action in relation to the information is frequently involved.	*I gathered the financial records.*	*I sorted the cookies and filled out the form.*	*I got together a list of schools, and sent out applications.*
Computing: Performing arithmetic operations and reporting on and/or carrying out a prescribed action in relation to them. Does not include counting.	*I figured out how much I would need.*	*I got an A and a B on my math report card.*	*I figured out much I would need for my student loan.*

4. Adult Unwaged Work Achievements	5. Adult Waged Work Achievements	6. Women Who Have Come Before Me	7. Miscellaneous
I wrote a resource manual for my PTA.	*I wrote a clerical manual.*	*I wrote poetry about my loss of my mother.*	
I set up the room and the meetings for my support group.	*I supervised the office staff.*	*I organized a trip to Chicago to trace my mother's life*	
I analyzed how much the housework could be shared by the whole family.	*I streamlined the operation at work.*	*I pored over my mother's college record and decided I wanted a college degree at my mother's school.*	*I tried out different sports before I took up yoga.*
I made grocery lists and menus.	*I took notes for the meeting, and distributed them.*	*I got together a list of schools and sent out applications while hoping to go to her school.*	*I read books, and watched video tapes on yoga before I started classes.*
I balanced the the checkbook.	*I balanced the the office checkbook.*	*I made a budget for my educational expenses.*	*I saved money out of the food budget to pay for classes.*

(continued on next page)

(continued from previous page)

My Achievement History	1. Saving My Own Life	2. Childhood Achievements	3. Adult Educational Achievements
Copying: Transcribing entering, or posting data.	*I made my own lists of addresses.*	*I copied the names of my of my favorite rock stars.*	*I posted my class schedule on the board.*
Comparing: Judging the readily observable functional, structural, or compositional characteristics (whether similar to or divergent from obvious standards) of data, people, or things.	*I noticed that other people did not have bruises.*	*My handwriting looks pretty good when compared to hers.*	*When I copied my friend's biology notes, I saw that hers were better than mine.*

4. Adult Unwaged Work Achievements	5. Adult Waged Work Achievements	6. Women Who Have Come Before Me	7. Miscellaneous
I did the posting in the books for my "husband's" business.	*I posted the accounts receivable.*	*I copied a list of my mother's courses and grades into my journal.*	*I made copies of yoga drawings into my journal.*
I looked at magazines to figure out how to decorate the apartment.	*I proofed the letter.*	*I observed the behaviors of other mothers and daughters.*	*I noticed that people who came to class frequently were quite imber.*

MY DATA SKILLS CHART

DATA: Information, knowledge, and conceptions, related to data, people, or things, obtained by observation, investigation, interpretation, visualization, and mental creation. Data are intangible and include numbers, words, symbols, ideas, concepts, and oral verbalization.

My Achievement History	1. Saving My Own Life	2. Childhood Achievements	3. Adult Educational Achievements
Synthesizing: Integrating analyses of data to discover facts concepts or interpretation. and/or develop knowledge			
Coordinating: Determining time, place, and sequence of operations or actions to be taken on the basis of analyzing data; executing determinations and/or reporting on events.			
Analyzing: Examining and evaluating data Presenting alternative actions in relation to the evaluation is frequently involved.			
Compiling: Gathering, collating, or classifying information about data, people, or things. Reporting and/or carrying out a prescribed action in relation to the information is frequently involved.			
Computing: Performing arithmetic operations and reporting on and/or carrying out a prescribed action in relation to them. Does not include counting			

4. Adult Unwaged Work Achievements	5. Adult Waged Achievements	6. Women Who Have Come Before Me	7. Miscellaneous

(continued on next page)

(continued from previous page)

My Achievement History	1. Saving My Own Life	2. Childhood Achievements	3. Adult Educational Achievements
Copying: Transcribing, entering, or posting data.			
Comparing: Judging the readily observable functional, structural, or characteristics (whether similar to or divergent from obvious standards) of data, people, or things.			

4. Adult Unwaged Work Achievements	5. Adult Waged Achievements	6. Women Who Have Come Before Me	7. Miscellaneous

TIP

Look for the patterns in your *Data Skills Chart.* The *Sample Data Skills Chart* indicates that similar skills or functions were used to perform waged and unwaged work (e.g., I balanced the check book. I balanced the office checkbook). The *Sample Data Skills Chart* also has blank spaces. That is, Synthesizing and Coordinating Skills were *not* used for Miscellaneous category. Learning yoga was a simple pleasure, and did not involve teaching or working with others. You may have blank spaces in your *Data Skills Chart* too. This is okay.

SAMPLE PEOPLE SKILLS CHART

People: Human Beings: Also animals dealt with on an individual basis as if they were human.

My Achievement History	1. Saving My Own Life	2. Childhood Achievements	3. Adult Education Achievements
Mentoring: Dealing with individuals in terms of their total personality in order to advise, counsel, and/or guide them with regard to problems that may be resolved by legal, scientific, clinical, spiritual, and/or other professional principles.	*I helped my husband with the divorce so I could be free.*	*My dog was my best friend.*	*I took parenting skills classes, and practiced with my kids.*
Negotiating: Exchanging ideas, information, and opinions with others to formulate policies and programs and/or arrive jointly at decisions, conclusions, or solutions.	*I worked closely with the attorney in making decisions about the divorce.*		*I got Fs removed from my transcripts by explaining the dynamics of battering to the Dean.*
Instructing: Teaching subject matter to others, or training others (including animals) through explanation, demonstration, and supervised practice, or making recommendations on the basis of technical disciplines.	*I trained my attorney about the dynamics of battering.*	*I trained my dog to do tricks.*	*I led groups for volunteers at the shelter, and got college credit for it.*
Supervising: Determining or interpreting work procedures for a group of workers, assigning specific duties to them, maintaining harmonious relations among them, and promoting efficiency. A variety of responsibilities is involved in this function.	*I explained the courtroom to my kids, and supervised their attendance throughout the trial.*	*I was in charge of my dog.*	*I supervised children as part of my internship as a teacher's aide.*
Diverting: Amusing others, usually through the medium of stage, screen, television, or radio.	*I slept with my husband in order to prevent him from beating my child.*	*I put on shows in the backyard.*	*I told jokes in class.*

4. Adult Unwaged Work Achievements	5. Adult Waged Work Achievements	6. Women Who Have Come Before Me	7. Miscellaneous
I raised my children by myself.		*My aunt is an attorney for battered women.*	*The kids in the neighborhood came to me to talk about their problems.*
I negotiated childcare duties with my new partner.	*I worked as the union steward.*	*She is known for coming up with great child custody solutions*	*I got two gang leaders to talk to each other.*
I trained the new volunteers to close up the office.	*I showed new people how to assemble the part.*	*My aunt trains volunteers at the shelter to write temporary restraining orders.*	*I trained them in saying "I" when using feeling statements.*
On my day at school as a parent volunteer, the kids get along.	*I became the lead person on my assembly line.*	*My aunt has three attorneys and four paralegals working for her.*	*I got them to agree to meet only under my eye.*
I directed the class sing-along.		*She is amazing in the courtroom.*	*I make jokes with the kids when they feel bad.*

(continued on next page)

(continued from previous page)

My Achievement History	1. Saving My Own Life	2. Childhood Achievements	3. Adult Education Achievements
Persuading: Influencing others in favor of a product, service, or point of view.	*I talked the would-be rapist into letting me go.*	*I sold neighbors girl scout cookies.*	*I gave speeches on rape in my sociology class.*
Speaking-Signaling: Talking with and/or signaling people to convey or exchange information. Includes giving assignments and/or directions to helpers or assistants.	*I arranged signals with my neighbor to call the police when the beatings were really bad.*	*I got a girl scout badge in the use of nautical flags.*	*I assigned the work tasks in my group project at school.*
Serving: Attending to the needs or requests of people or animals or the expressed or implicit wishes of people. Immediate response is involved.	*I made dinner for my father before I ran away.*	*I did all the dishes.*	*I studied patient care.*
Taking Instructions-Helping: Attending to work assignment instructions or orders of a supervisor.	*I did exactly what the police told me to do.*	*I helped the teacher with after school clean-up.*	*I followed classroom assignments exactly.*

4. Adult Unwaged Work Achievements	5. Adult Waged Work Achievements	6. Women Who Have Come Before Me	7. Miscellaneous
I convinced them to sing Jingle Bells.	*I got them to use my idea.*	*Juries usually agree with her.*	*I insisted that they leave their weapons outside the door of my house.*
The kids knew when I raised my eyes that they should hide.	*People waited for my signal to shut down the line.*	*I used the gang signals I knew in order to get the kids to talk to me.*	*She could get information into her hand in the courtroom with a signal to her paralegal.*
I watered and fed all the animals.	*I got a job as a ranch hand.*	*My aunt also served turkey at Thanksgiving.*	*I fed the kids cookies.*
I followed the instructions on how to use the milking machine.	*The boss taught me how to use the milking machine.*	*My aunt learned how to serve properly by following instructions from the paid staff at the Mission.*	*I followed the directions given to me by the youth counselor.*

MY PEOPLE SKILLS CHART

My Achievement History	1. Saving My Own Life	2. Childhood Achievements	3. Adult Educational Achievements
Mentoring: Dealing with individuals in terms of their total personality in order to advise, counsel, and/or guide them with regard to problems that may be resolved by legal, scientific, clinical, spiritual, and/or other professional principles			
Negotiating: Exchanging ideas, information, and opinions with others to formulate policies and programs and/or arrive jointly at decisions, conclusions, or solutions.			
Instructing: Teaching subject matter to others, or training others (including animals) through explanation, demonstration, and supervised practice, or making recommendations on the basis of technical disciplines.			
Supervising: Determining or interpreting work procedures for a group of workers, assigning specific duties to them, maintaining harmonious relations among them, and promoting efficiency. A variety of responsibilities is involved in this function.			
Diverting: Amusing others, usually through the medium of stage, screen, television, or radio.			

4. Adult Unwaged Work Achievements	5. Adult Waged Work Achievements	6. Women Who Have Come Before Me	7. Miscellaneous

(continued on next page)

(continued from previous page)

My Achievement History	1. Saving My Own Life	2. Childhood Achievements	3. Adult Education Achievements
Persuading: Influencing others in favor of a product, service, or point of view.			
Speaking-Signaling: Talking with and/or signaling people to convey or exchange information. Includes giving assignments and/or directions to helpers or assistants.			
Serving: Attending to the needs or requests of people or animals or the expressed or implicit wishes of people. Immediate response is involved.			
Taking Instructions-Helping: Attending to work assignment instructions or orders of a supervisor.			

4. Adult Unwaged Work Achievements	5. Adult Waged Work Achievements	6. Women Who Have Come Before Me	7. Miscellaneous

SAMPLE THINGS SKILLS CHART

THINGS: Inanimate objects as distinguished from human beings, substances or materials; and machines, tools, equipment, work aids, and products. A thing is tangible and has shape, form, and other physical characteristics.

My Achievement History	1. Saving My Own Life	2. Childhood Achievements	3. Adult Educational Achievements
Setting Up: Preparing machines (or equipment) for operation by planning order of successive machine operations, installing and adjusting tools and other machine components, adjusting the position of the work piece or material, setting controls, and verifying accuracy of machine capabilities, properties of materials, and shop practices. Uses tools, equipment, and work aids, such as precision gauges and measuring instruments. Workers who set up one or a number of machine for other workers or who set up and personally operate a variety of machines are included here.			*I set up the de-burring machine for other students at my technical school.*
Precision Working: Using body members and/or tools or work aids to work, move, guide, or place objects or materials in situations where ultimate responsibility for the attainment of standards occurs and selections of appropriate tools, objects, or materials, and the adjustment of the tool to the task require exercise of considerable judgment.	*I made gourmet dinners so he wouldn't beat me.*	*I made my own paper dolls and their clothes.*	*I adjusted the machines as needed at technical school.*
Operating-Controlling: Starting, stopping, controlling, and adjusting the progress of machines or equipment. Operating machines involves setting up and adjusting the machine or material(s) as the work progresses.	*I used the juicer to prepare fresh vegetable and fruit juices, and baby food as my husband demanded.*		*I ran my own machine at the technical school.*

4. Adult Unwaged Work Achievements	5. Adult Waged Work Achievements	6. Women Who Have Come Before Me	7. Miscellaneous
		The artist, Judy Chicago, directed the firing of the porcelain plates for The Dinner Party.	*I set up the drill presses for my father in his home workshop.*
		Chicago learned and used china painting techniques for The Dinner Party.	*I measured all the pieces of wood in my father's home workshop.*
I always took charge of the copy machine at the shelter as part of my volunteer work.	*I was the key operator at work for the copy machine.*		*I used the staple gun under my father's supervision.*

(continued on next page)

(continued from previous page)

My Achievement History	1. Saving My Own Life	2. Childhood Achievements	3. Adult Educational Achievements
Driving-Operating: Starting, stopping, and controlling the actions of machines or equipment for which a course must by steered or which must be guided to control the movement of things or people for a variety of purposes.	*I drove the getaway car on the freeway to get to the shelter.*	*I drove the car when my Dad was drunk when I was only nine years old.*	*I obtained my truck driver's license through truck driving school.*
Manipulating: Using body members, tools, or special devices to work, move, guide, or place objects or materials. Involves some latitude for judgment with regard to precision attained and selecting appropriate tool, object, or material, although this is readily manifest.	*I learned how to put the distributor cap back in the car after my husband had removed it.*	*I built my own dollhouse.*	*At truck driver school, I learned how to change a tire, check the oil, lube the vehicle.*
Tending: Starting, stopping, and observing the functioning of machines and equipment. Involves materials or controls of the machine, such as changing guides, adjusting timers and temperature gauges, turning valves to allow flow of materials, and flipping switches in response to lights. Little judgment is involved in making these adjustment.		*I had a toy train which I operated on tracks around my bedroom.*	*I also took a course in tanker truck operation.*
Feeding-Offbearing: Inserting, throwing, dumping, or placing materials in or removing them from machines or equipment which are automatic or tended or operated by other workers.		*I fed the leaves and branches into the shredder while my Mom operated it.*	*I learned to use automatic pallets as part of my truck driver training.*
Handling: Using body members, handtools, and/or special devices to work, move, or carry objects or materials. Involves little or no latitude for judgment with regard to attainment of standards or in selecting appropriate tool, object, or materials.	*I packed the toys, the books, and our clothes for use at the shelter.*	*I did the dishes regularly.*	*I learned the best way to load and unload a truck.*

4. Adult Unwaged Work Achievements	5. Adult Waged Work Achievements	6. Women Who Have Come Before Me	7. Miscellaneous
I was a volunteer driver.	*I drove the truck across country.*		
I helped paint the new house.	*I worked on the assembly line.*	*Chicago colored in all the cartoons she had created for the weavers.*	*I painted the new rape crisis center office.*
I kept the furnace going all winter.	*I ran the copier.*	*Chicago used her own paint mixing machine.*	*I ran the fax machine.*
I used the shredder to clean up the lawn.	*I used the shredder at the office.*		*I used an old fashion wringer washing machine.*
I took all of the shredded material to the community garden.	*I stocked the grocery shelves.*	*Chicago handled brushes, plates, books, alter clothes, spools, paint cans, and thousands of items needed to create The Dinner Party.*	*I also hung clothes on a clothsline.*

MY THINGS SKILLS CHART

THINGS: Inanimate objects as distinguished from human beings, substances or materials; and machines, tools, equipment, work aids, and products. A thing is tangible and has shape, form, and other physical characteristics.

My Achievement History	1. Saving My Own Life	2. Childhood Achievements	3. Adult Educational Achievements
Setting Up: Preparing machines (or equipment) for operation by planning order of successive machine operations, installing and adjusting tools and other machine components, adjusting the position of the work piece or material, setting controls, and verifying accuracy of machine capabilities, properties of materials, and shop practices. Uses tools, equipment, and work aids, such as precision gauges and measuring instruments. Workers who set up one or a number of machine for other workers or who set up and personally operate a variety of machines are included here.			
Precision Working: Using body members and/ or tools or work aids to work, move, guide, or place objects or materials in situations where ultimate responsibility for the attainment of standards occurs and selections of appropriate tools, objects, or materials, and the adjustment of the tool to the task require exercise of considerable judgment.			
Operating-Controlling: Starting, stopping, controlling, and adjusting the progress of machines or equipment. Operating machines involves setting up and adjusting the machine or material(s) as the work progresses.			

4. Adult Unwaged Work Achievements	5. Adult Waged Work Achievements	6. Women Who Have Come Before Me	7. Miscellaneous

(continued on next page)

(continued from previous page)

My Achievement History	1. Saving My Own Life	2. Childhood Achievements	3. Adult Educational Achievements
Driving-Operating: Starting, stopping, and controlling the actions of machines or equipment for which a course must by steered or which must be guided to control the movement of things or people for a variety of purposes.			
Manipulating: Using body members, tools, or special devices to work, move, guide, or place objects or materials. Involves some latitude for judgment with regard to precision attained and selecting appropriate tool, object, or material, although this is readily manifest.			
Tending: Starting, stopping, and observing the functioning of machines and equipment. Involves materials or controls of the machine, such as changing guides, adjusting timers and temperature gauges, turning valves to allow flow of materials, and flipping switches in response to lights. Little judgment is involved in making these adjustment.			
Feeding-Offbearing: Inserting, throwing, dumping, or placing materials in or removing them from machines or equipment which are automatic or tended or operated by other workers.			
Handling: Using body members, handtools, and/or special devices to work, move, or carry objects or materials. Involves little or no latitude for judgment with regard to attainment of standards or in selecting appropriate tool, object, or materials.			

4. Adult Unwaged Work Achievements	5. Adult Waged Work Achievements	6. Women Who Have Come Before Me	7. Miscellaneous

---

TIP

Remember, you may or may not have used all of the worker functions listed above. Most of us are not skilled at everything. For example, you probably did not know how to drive a car when you were a child. Therefore, you will probably not be completing the *Driving-Operating* section under Childhood Achievements. That's okay. In these exercises, what you do not complete will be just as important as what you do complete, but that discussion is reserved for the next chapter. You may also find yourself remembering details you did not write down in the *Making Your Work Visible* chapter. That's good. You may wish to add detail to that chapter now. Remember, most of us survivors either are, or have been, members of the If-I-Can-Do-It-It-Must-Not-Be-Much-Club. We tend to discount the quality and quantity of our skills. These exercises allow us to practice thinking and talking about our skills.

You may now resign from the If-I-Can-Do-It-It-Must-Not-Be-Much-Club because you now have a record of your transferable skills. And not only that, it's official, because this record, this document you have created, is based on the United States government's Department of Labor's official description of worker functions: *The Dictionary of Occupational Titles*. This book uses these worker functions to analyze the more than 12,000 jobs listed. In other words, you now know what skills you presently have which could be matched to more than 12,000 jobs!!!

In the next chapter, *Understanding Your Vocational Impairment*, we will be pulling together all of the work you have completed so far. You now have tools. You have made your own worklife visible. You understand your transferable skills. You are on your way through the flower or moving into the reality of your waged and unwaged worklife. The process of understanding your vocational impairment is necessary to move to the last section of the Workbook. *The Plan – Reweaving Your Won Life and Work*. Like all weavers, you must gather the strands together before you can see the pattern, heal the damage, design and weave a new life.

nine

---

understanding your
vocational impairment

*It seems to me that growth takes place by starting where we really
are and moving on. We women have spent much of our time hiding
who we are, because we have been made to feel ashamed.*

Judy Chicago, 1979, p. 114

The purpose of this chapter is to synthesize what has come before. The chapters,
*Naming the Trauma, Re-Claiming My Innocent Body, Making Your Work Visible,
and Analyzing, Respecting, and Celebrating Your Work*, have been what Chicago
describes as "starting where we really
are." This chapter completes that process so that we can get to the next step,
which is "moving on."

We will return to *Naming the
Trauma* so that we can identify the
negative worker traits which have created vocational barriers or impairment
in your waged and unwaged worklife.
We will re-examine *Re-Claiming My
Innocent Body* for your ability to meet
physical demands in work or the physical limitations which may preclude
you from certain jobs. We will summarize your educational attainment
level by looking once again at *Making Your Work Visible*. We will identify some of your important transferable skills by revisiting *Analyzing,
Respecting, and Celebrating Your
Work*.

TIP

If this chapter brings up feelings and/or thoughts of shame,
go to the chapter, *Overcoming
Verbal-Emotional Abuse*, in order
to create an affirmation which
will assist you in doing the work of
this chapter. A suggested affirmation is: *I, (name) am proud of the
work I've done.* Self-forgiveness
work might also be important
here since we may feel overcome by shame at some of our
negative health habits (substance abuse) or post-traumatic
stress disorder symptoms (anger
inappropriately expressed). The
discovery of our own innocence
allows us to move on from guilt
and shame so that we can do our
work. The suggested affirmation
here is, *I, (name) am innocent
and I forgive myself completely.*

a negative worker traits analysis

Crying jags, depressions, and self-deprecating remarks were rampant. The women weren't at all confident that they could make the change. Many of them were extremely angry at me for making demands upon them that they were afraid they couldn't meet.

Judy Chicago, 1979, p. 85

Worker traits are traits which are used in connection with a work activity. For example, a musician requires both a good sense of pitch and fine finger dexterity (traits) to play a piece of music by ear without error (skill). A positive attitude may be an important worker trait for a nurse. A well groomed appearance is a positive worker trait for receptionists and television news journalists. There are also negative worker traits, and these can evolve as a result of traumatic abuse. In fact, the post-traumatic stress disorder (PTSD) symptoms we explored in the chapter, *Naming the Trauma,* can also be defined as negative worker traits. For example, irritability and/or outbursts of anger are both symptoms of PTSD and negative worker traits since such behaviors are inappropriate in the waged work world and in the unwaged worklife of raising children. Supervisors or mentors are unlikely to tolerate such behaviors and co-workers are not likely to become workplace friends. In the unwaged

> **TIP**
> In choosing anger and/or irritability as my example of a negative worker trait, I am not attempting to reinforce what Heilbrun (1988, p. 13) describes as "And, above all other prohibitions, what has been forbidden to women is anger, together with the open admission of the desire for power and control over one's life." Rather, I am suggesting that anger inappropriately expressed (e.g., to one's children or a supervisor or mentor instead of to the rapist, the molester, the battering partner) is not in your self-interest. In fact, my favorite line in the Sally Field and Joanne Woodward film of the novel *Sibyl* is when Joanne Woodward's character, the therapist, tells Sibyl (Sally Field) that "anger is your friend." I agree. Anger appropriately expressed is a good friend, a source of motivation, energy, and inspiration. Learning the difference is a good thing to practice with your therapist or your support group.

work world of parenting, children may carry the anger expressed toward them into their educational lives with similar results from teachers and schoolmates.

The following list was developed by examining the *Possible Vocational Impairment* categories under the *Naming the Trauma Exercises* for the PTSD and complex posttraumatic stress disorder (CPTSD) symptoms from the chapter, *Naming the Trauma.* My suggestion is that you look at the work you completed in that chapter, and make any additions to the list which seem appropriate.

TIP

Remember, the purpose of this list is to help you move on by understanding where you are now. With this information, you will be able to develop the best plan for yourself in your life and work.

A List of Negative Worker Traits Resulting From Traumatic Abuse

NEGATIVE WORKER TRAITS	YES	MAYBE	NO
Difficulty in learning at school.			
Difficulty in learning on the job.			
Difficulty in learning new tasks.			
Lack of mental clarity.			
Inability to concentrate or focus.			
Distracted by flashbacks.			
Distracted by illusions or hallucinations.			
Distracted by strong feelings.			
Difficulty in socializing with others.			
Difficulty in being in places which remind me of the trauma(s).			
Difficulty in functioning on the anniversary(ies) of the trauma(s).			
Mental fatigue.			
Inability to relax and let my creative self solve problems.			
Inability to leave the house.			
Ability to only be in certain places at certain times of the day.			
Inability to drive at all because of fear.			
Inability to drive on the freeway because of fear.			
Avoidance of activities which may involve self-expression such as singing, dancing, painting, writing.			
Inability to remember feelings and ideas.			
A lack of interest in things generally.			
An inability to guarantee punctuality.			
An inability to guarantee the keeping of appointments at all.			

A List of Negative Worker Traits Resulting From Traumatic Abuse (continued)

NEGATIVE WORKER TRAITS	YES	MAYBE	NO
An inability to get to work on time.			
An inability to get to school on time.			
High absenteeism at work.			
High absenteeism at school.			
An inability to plan for the future.			
A limited ability to even have a vision of a long range future in career or family life.			
An inability to make commitments.			
Withdrawn from others.			
Limited social skills in the workplace.			
Limited parenting skills.			
No pleasure in work.			
No pleasure in learning or school.			
No pleasure in family life.			
No expectation of living very long.			
Irritability.			
Outbursts of anger.			
Lack of self-confidence.			
Suspicious. Always on the lookout.			
Fearful. Easily frightened.			
Chronic illness.			
Many minor illnesses.			
Substance abuse.			
No waged work history.			
Limited waged work history.			
No understanding of the social aspects of waged work.			
No training in housework.			
No training in self care skills.			
Criminal record.			
In physical pain.			
In mental pain.			
No support systems.			
Isolated.			
Thinking about suicide.			
Sexually vulnerable.			
Sexually impulsive.			
Taking risks in sexual behaviors.			

A List of Negative Worker Traits Resulting From Traumatic Abuse (continued)

NEGATIVE WORKER TRAITS	YES	MAYBE	NO
Leaving my body.			
Disassociating/disappearing.			
Thinking about the trauma(s) all the time.			
Shame, guilt, stigma.			
Believe I was born to be a prostitute.			
Helpless and paralyzed.			
Feel stupid.			
Feel crazy.			
Believe I have no rights.			
Loss of name.			
Fearful that employer will tell perpetrator where I am.			
Waiting for perpetrator to tell me what to do.			
Expect to be moving all the time.			
Can't have an achievement level higher than my perpetrator(s).			
If I have my own money, I'll be hurt.			
Expect to be sexually harassed on the job.			
Expect to be sexually harassed at school.			
Don't trust anybody.			
Don't protect myself at work.			
Usually underemployed for my educational level or my intellectual level.			
Loss of faith in a higher power.			
Nothing matters anyway.			
No passion in my life, my work.			
My children don't matter either.			

Other Negative Worker Traits I Identified

_____

_____

_____

_____

_____

_____

_____

_____

_____

_____

_____

This list helps us to understand why even some highly educated survivors are unable to hold a job, or advance in their careers. Or why apparently privileged middle class white women with college educations are working as motel maids. Or why some survivors may do well at work, but are cranky and impossible at home. Or why some survivors who have the ability to benefit from further education cannot step foot on a college campus. Or why some women think they have no right to protest sexual harassment. Or why some traumatic abuse survivors cannot take intellectual or career risks even when such risks may be in their best interest. Or why survivors who were brutalized as children by beatings and neglect may not grasp the importance of good hygiene, grooming, proper rest, and nutrition for themselves or their children. Skill development and educational attainment, by themselves, are not sufficient for a fully developed work and family life.

A Summary of My Most Common Negative Worker Traits

_____

_____

_____

_____

_____

_____

_____

_____

_____

_____

_____

_____

_____

_____

_____

_____

_____

_____

_____

_____

In the next section of the Workbook, *The Plan–Re-Weaving Your Own Life and Work*, we will explore options for the healing and transformation of your negative worker traits. Often vocational planning excludes such healing, and focuses only on skill training of some sort. On the other hand, psychologists and psychotherapists often neglect skill training and intellectual development when guiding abuse survivors through a recovery process. In this process of *moving through the flower* a holistic approach is taken—mind, soul, and body—the whole person, the whole woman is affirmed.

my physical work capacity

> *There was a lot of resentment about the demands that were being made: to be there every day; to do unaccustomed physical labor, which many of them were unaccustomed to; to push beyond their emotional and physical limits. They complained of being tired, of having aches and pains. Some women were extremely concerned about their bodies, in an overprotective way. They had been raised to see their bodies as an important aspect of their attractiveness. Whereas men generally see their bodies as objects to be built up, strengthened, used, and exercised, women are often horrified about developing muscles that will defeminize them, are afraid of strenuous activities, and are anxious about every little discomfort. Admittedly men carry their disregard for the limits of human strength to unreasonable lengths, but women too often carry their self-protectiveness beyond a healthy point.*
>
> Judy Chicago, 1979, p. 106

In my career as a vocational rehabilitation counselor, I have had women get furious with me for suggesting that they might wish to explore nontraditional careers in the construction trades. This was true even for women whose interest inventory results indicated that they had not the slightest interest in the occupations usually set aside for women, such as the service occupations (nursing, teaching) and clerical work. Formerly battered women were particularly resistant to my suggestions even though their transition from the violent home, to the domestic violence shelter system, to having to make do on welfare checks (in an apartment located in crime ridden areas of Los Angeles) indicated that a good paying job might be a way out of a no-win economic pattern.

Chicago's analysis of her women students' resistance to physical work offers an explanation for the reaction of the traumatic abuse survivors. Traumatic abuse survivors may have even a greater investment in clinging to traditional ideas of femininity than female college students, since part of the abuse experience may have been the development of a deeply hurtful negative thought: *I am a defective woman*. Women with physical disabilities understand this thought with painful clarity. They have to endure the daily onslaught of what bodily perfection is for women in our culture. A woman with a pre-existing physical disability who also experiences traumatic abuse may have absorbed this negative thought to a level of utter anguish. A woman whose physical disability resulted from traumatic abuse may be completely convinced that *I am a defective woman.*

Therefore, my naive suggestion that such women might want to take part in the building of the Century Freeway in the heart of Los Angeles County was greeted with horror, astonishment, and rage. Was I trying to help formerly battered women become even more defective? Less feminine? Less attractive to men? No woman actually said these things to me, of course, and so it has taken me years to understand their reaction. I suspect that the well-meaning folks in the personnel office for the Century Freeway are still trying to figure out why women haven't been flocking to their doors.

> **TIP**
> The conscious breathing exercise described in the chapter, *Re-Claiming My Innocent Body*, is recommended now. You may find yourself disappearing or disassociating as you move through this portion of the work. The slow and easy inhalation and exhalation of your breath will give you the nourishment and strength to continue. Take at least three slow and easy breaths.

> **TIP**
> The use of the affirmation process described in the chapter, *Overcoming Verbal-Emotional Abuse*, is also recommended now. A suggested affirmation is: *I, (name) am a whole, healthy, and perfect woman.*

The Dictionary of Occupational Titles categorizes the physical demands of the more than 12,000 jobs it lists as sedentary, light, medium, heavy, and very heavy work. This reference work and the Social Security Administration, Office of Hearings and Appeals (1990, February) also define work by exertional activities, exertional levels, exertional limitations, and nonexertional impairments and limitations.

Sedentary Work is lifting 10 pounds maximum and occasionally lifting and/or carrying such articles as dockets, ledgers, and small tools. Although a sedentary job is defined as one which involves sitting, a certain amount of walking and standing is often necessary in carrying out job duties. Jobs are sedentary if walking and standing are required only occasionally and other sedentary criteria are met.

Light Work is lifting 20 pounds maximum with frequent lifting and/or carrying of objects weighing up to 10 pounds. Even thought the weight lifted may be only a negligible amount, a job is in this category when it requires walking or standing to a significant degree, or when it involves sitting most of the time with a degree of pushing and pulling of arm and/or leg controls.

Medium Work is lifting 50 pounds maximum with frequent lifting and/or carrying of objects weighing up to 50 pounds.

Heavy Work is lifting 100 pounds maximum with frequent lifting and/or carrying of objects weighing up to 50 pounds.

Very Heavy Work is lifting objects in excess of 100 pounds with frequent lifting and/or carrying of objects weighing 50 pounds or more.

The categories of heavy and very heavy work may be what Chicago has in mind when she writes, "Admittedly men carry their disregard for the limits of human strength to unreasonable lengths..." In fact, women's entry into occupations dominated by men has been good for men and women, since the lifting requirements in these jobs tend to move from heavy and very heavy work to medium work when women enter the occupation. One example of this is women's entry into telephone installation jobs. Tools, tool belts, and the equipment men and women now use when climbing telephone poles are now lighter and easier to handle.

The human spine (male or female) is simply not designed to lift and carry excessive weights. This is a truth which can be attested to by any orthopedic surgeon, workers' compensation claims examiner, vocational rehabilitation counselor, and heavy construction worker. Chicago's point that the physical demands of the workplace need some sort of gender balance in terms of reasonableness may be the answer to the costly results of back injuries in our society. This reasonableness needs to extend into the home as well, where women can be found performing heavy and very heavy lifting in the care of children, persons with disabilities, or elderly parents.

The seesaw between excessive exertion and overprotectiveness of one's body has a curiously parallel relationship to the denial process experienced by traumatic abuse survivors. For example, two co-researchers in *Making the Connections: Women, Work & Abuse*, reported that they ignored their bodies' pain to the extent that one required surgery and the other delayed medical treatment. And as we have seen, overprotectiveness of one's body is also a form of denial demonstrated by women when they have to face the gendered workplace. The extreme segregation of the workplace by gender, or the tying of certain kinds of work to sexual potency, in our culture leads to strange distortions in our thinking about work and sexuality. Therefore when you complete the *My Physical Work Capacity* analysis worksheet, aim for moderation in your responses. Be neither tough nor tender. Be realistic. Be reasonable.

Exertional Activity is one of the primary strength activities (walk, stand, sit, lift, carry, push, pull) which defines a level of work.

Exertional Level is a work classification defining the functional requirements of work in terms of the primary strength activities required (sedentary, light, medium, heavy and very heavy work).

Exertional Limitation is an impairment-caused restriction which affects capability to perform an exertional activity (sitting, standing, walking, pushing, pulling, lifting, and/or carrying).

Nonexertional Impairment is an impairment which does not directly affect the ability to sit, stand, walk, lift, carry, push or pull. This includes impairments which affect the mind, vision, hearing, speech, and use of the body to climb, balance, stoop, kneel, crouch, crawl, reach, handle, and use of the fingers for fine activities.

Nonexertional Limitation is an impairment-caused limitation of function which directly affects capability to perform work activities other than the primary strength activities.

Perhaps the development of the video display terminal work station provides us with the most fascinating example of the gendered workplace, and how the gendering of the workplace also affects the exertional and nonexertional physical demands of the workers within it. Before the computer revolution, secretaries (female) sat (exertional activity) in secretarial chairs which were designed for the female body. The executives (male), for whom these female clerical workers typed (nonexertional activity), sat (exertional activity) in executive chairs which were designed for the male body.

Havoc ensued when the computer display terminal showed up on female and male desks. I found myself with 250 pound industrially injured male workers at office furniture stores trying to find chairs that would not collapse under their weights while they tried to make big hands and fingers operate (nonexertional activity) a computer keyboard. The executive chairs didn't work very well because they were not designed to be pulled under a desk for typing on a computer keyboard or typewriter. An industrially injured male with a bad back didn't have a prayer in surviving in such a chair anyway. He needed more support for his back. And besides, the executive chairs, with their arms and leather upholstery, were more expensive. No insurance company wanted to spring for a $500 chair. In those days, the poor guys usually ended up with a cheap, and badly designed, executive chair. As the computer revolution progressed through the 80s, women began to report pain in their wrists and arms. An epidemic of carpal tunnel syndrome swept the country, and is still with us. In the 90s, we have secretarial chairs with arms (to take the strain of the weight of the arms off the neck and back and to help in keeping the wrists level while typing on the keyboard); chairs with adjustable back support (to make the exertional activity of sitting not so strenuous); and work station design for lighting, including non-glare screens for display monitors (improvements to the nonexertional activity of seeing). Executives and professionals (now male and female), in the meantime, are still sitting in executive chairs at executive desks with a computer display terminal perched in one corner. I found a female attorney with telephone books under her feet, entering data into her computer (exertional and nonexertional activity). "Does your back hurt?" I asked, eyeing her executive chair which had no adjustable back support. "All the time," she replied.

The computer revolution has turned the gendered office workplace on its head. As the dust settles, we seem to be left with class issues. That is, executives and professionals don't want to give up their status symbols of executive chairs and desks even though more and more workers, at every level, are working at video display terminal workstations. My reason for this digression on computer workstations is that the women I've counseled in workers' compensation systems, with carpal tunnel syndrome and other cumulative trauma injuries resulting from the so-called *nonexertional activities* of typing on computer keyboards, display some of the same symptoms of traumatic abuse survivors. I think this is because, like trauma survivors, women with carpal tunnel syndrome injuries have a hard time being taken seriously, and so by the time an injured woman is referred for vocational rehabilitation services, she has had the experience of being disbelieved. She may have been told her problem is psychological. She may have been fired from her job Or, she may have landed in the clutches of one or more orthopedist and undergone one or more surgeries which have not given her any relief from the pain in her wrists and arms. She may be unable to cook dinner for her family because she cannot pick up a sauce pan without dropping it.

Given the powerful impulse of traumatic abuse survivors to deny pain in their bodies and injury to their bodies, and given the fact that the so called *nonexertional activity* of computer keyboard typing is producing an epidemic level of injury in clerical workers, who are mostly women; *traumatic abuse* survivors, who are also clerical workers, are at great risk for cumulative trauma injuries to their *wrists, arms, backs, necks.* Negative worker traits and/or posttraumatic stress disorder symptoms, such as *physical pain, lack of self confidence, belief that you have no rights, leaving the body, disassociating/disappearing,* all conspire to undermine the trauma survivor's ability to assert herself in the workplace by asking for a better chair, a no-glare screen, a desk at the right height.

The injuries which result from the static posture of sitting in front of a monitor while entering data by typing on a keyboard are cumulative in much the same way verbal-emotional abuse is cumulative. That is, the injury does not become noticeable the first time, or even the hundredth time. It is the constant and gradual accumulation of insults to heart, mind, and body which takes place moment by moment, hour by hour, day by day, week by week, month by month, and even year by year. Finally, the pain is ever present in the wrists, and in the heart and soul.

Therefore when you complete the exertional and nonexertional portions of the *My Physical Capacity Work* analysis, do not discount nor deny these apparently unimportant physical demands. You, and all trauma survivors, deserve a comfortable, pain-free work life. And, as usual, an ounce of prevention (comparatively nonexertional) is worth a pound of cure (overwhelmingly exertional).

SAMPLE PHYSICAL WORK CAPACITY

I Can Now Perform The Following Lifting Activities

Frequency (8 hour shift)	Yes? No?	Occasional (0 to 3 hrs)	Frequent (3 to 6 hrs)	Continuous?	Intermittent?	How Many Rest Breaks?
Sedentary Work (lifting 10 pounds maximum and occasionally lifting and/or carrying such articles as dockets, ledgers, and small tools.)	yes	yes	yes	yes	yes	at least 2 with lunch
Light Work (lifting 20 pounds maximum with frequent lifting and/or carrying of objects weighing up to 10 pounds.)	yes	yes	yes	no	yes	at least 2 with lunch
Medium Work (lifting 50 pounds maximum with frequent lifting and/or carrying of objects weighing up to 50 pounds.)	yes	yes	no	no	yes	at least 2 with lunch
Heavy Work (lifting 100 pounds maximum with frequent lifting and/or carrying of objects weighing up to 50 pounds.)	no	no	no	no	no	
Very Heavy Work (lifting objects in excess of 100 pounds with frequent lifting and/or carrying of objects weighing 50 pounds or more.)	no	no	no	no	no	

MY PHYSICAL WORK CAPACITY

I CAN NOW PERFORM THE FOLLOWING LIFTING ACTIVITIES

Frequency (8 hour shift)	Yes? No?	Occasional (0 to 3 hrs)	Frequent (3 to 6 hrs)	Continuous? Breaks?	Intermittent?	How Many Rest
Sedentary Work (lifting 10 pounds maximum and occasionally lifting and/or carrying such articles as dockets, ledgers, and small tools.)						
Light Work (lifting 20 pounds maximum with frequent lifting and/or carrying of objects weighing up to 10 pounds.)						
Medium Work (lifting 50 pounds maximum with frequent lifting and/or carrying of objects weighing up to 50 pounds.)						
Heavy Work (lifting 100 pounds maximum with frequent lifting and/or carrying of objects weighing up to 50 pounds.)						
Very Heavy Work (lifting objects in excess of 100 pounds with frequent lifting and/or carrying of objects weighing 50 pounds or more.)						

Sample Summary of Lifting Capacities & Limitations

As a middle-aged woman with a regular exercise program and minor orthopedic problems, my lifting capacities include the ability to do sedentary, light, and medium work with the appropriate coffee breaks and midday lunch hour. Except for sedentary work, I would find it difficult to do lifting on a continuous basis with no opportunity to perform other activities such as walking or sitting. My lifting limitations are no frequent lifting beyond 50 pounds. (Persons using wheelchairs, canes, walkers; and persons with orthopedic problems may have many lifting restrictions.)

My Summary of Lifting Capacities and Limitations

_____

_____

_____

_____

_____

_____

_____

_____

_____

_____

_____

SAMPLE PHYSICAL WORK CAPACITY continued...

I Can Now Perform The Following Exertional Activities

Frequency (8 hour shift)	Yes? No?	Occasional (0 to 3 hrs)	Frequent (3 to 6 hrs)	Continuous?	Intermittent?	How Many Rest Breaks?
Sitting	yes	yes	yes	no	yes	get up every hour
Walking	yes	yes	yes	yes	yes	every hour or two
Standing	yes	yes	yes	no	yes	every hour
Pushing	yes	yes	no	no	yes	every few minutes
Pulling	yes	yes	no	no	yes	every few minutes

Sample Summary of Exertional Activity Levels

I am able to perform all of these primary strength activities. My limitations are with pushing and pulling which could only be performed by me occasionally with frequent rest breaks. My lifting restrictions of no frequent lifting beyond 50 pounds means that if the item to be pushed or pulled weighs more than 50 pounds and is not on wheels or rollers, I would probably not be able to push or pull it at all. (Persons with orthopedic limitations may have many limitations with these exertional activities.)

MY PHYSICAL WORK CAPACITY continued...

I Can Now Perform The Following Exertional Activities

Frequency (8 hour shift)	Yes? No?	Occasional (0 to 3 hrs)	Frequent (3 to 6 hrs)	Continuous?	Intermittent?	How Many Rest Breaks?
Sitting						
Walking						
Standing						
Pushing						
Pulling						

My Summary of My Exertional Activity Levels

SAMPLE PHYSICAL WORK CAPACITY continued...

I Can Now Perform The Following Nonexertional Activities

Frequency (8 hour shift)	Yes? No?	Occasional (0 to 3 hrs)	Frequent (3 to 6 hrs)	Continuous?	Intermittent?	How Many Rest Breaks?
Seeing	yes	yes	yes	yes	yes	none
Hearing	yes	yes	yes	yes	yes	none
Speaking	yes	yes	yes	no	yes	maximum one hour

Sample Summary of Nonexertional Activity Levels

I am able to perform the activities of hearing, seeing, and speaking. I have found that continuous speaking is not possible for me however, since my voice gives out. (Persons with visual and hearing impairments may need to take frequent rest breaks if they are able to hear or see at all.)

MY PHYSICAL WORK CAPACITY continued...

I Can Now Perform The Following Nonexertional Activities

Frequency (8 hour shift)	Yes? No?	Occasional (0 to 3 hrs)	Frequent (3 to 6 hrs)	Continuous?	Intermittent?	How Many Rest Breaks?
Seeing						
Hearing						
Speaking						

My Summary of My Nonexertional Activity Levels

_____

_____

_____

_____

_____

_____

_____

_____

_____

SAMPLE PHYSICAL WORK CAPACITY continued...

I Am Able To Use My Body For The Following Nonexertional Activities

Frequency (8 hour shift)	Yes? No?	Occasional (0 to 3 hrs)	Frequent (3 to 6 hrs)	Continuous?	Intermittent?	How Many Rest Breaks?
Climbing	yes	yes	yes	no	yes	very often
Balancing	yes	yes	yes	yes	no	none
Stooping	yes	yes	no	no	yes	very often
Kneeling	yes	yes	no	no	yes	very often
Crouching	yes	yes	no	no	yes	very often
Crawling	yes	yes	no	no	yes	very often
Reaching	yes	yes	yes	no	yes	every few minutes
Handling (right hand)	yes	yes	yes	yes	yes	every hour
Handling (left hand)	yes	yes	yes	yes	yes	every 1/2 hour
Grasping (right hand)	yes	yes	no	no	yes	every few minutes
Grasping (left hand)	yes	yes	no	no	yes	every few minutes
Fine Manipulation with fingers (right hand)	yes	yes	yes	yes	yes	every hour
Fine Manipulation with fingers (left hand)	yes	yes	yes	yes	yes	every hour
Operate foot pedals (right foot)	yes	yes	yes	no	yes	every 3 to 4 hours
Operate foot pedals (left foot)	yes	yes	yes	no	yes	every 3 to 4 hours

MY PHYSICAL WORK CAPACITY continued...

I Am Able To Use My Body For The Following Nonexertional Activities

Frequency (8 hour shift)	Yes? No?	Occasional (0 to 3 hrs)	Frequent (3 to 6 hrs)	Continuous?	Intermittent?	How Many Rest Breaks?
Climbing						
Balancing						
Stooping						
Kneeling						
Crouching						
Crawling						
Reaching						
Handling (right hand)						
Handling (left hand)						
Grasping (right hand)						
Grasping (left hand)						
Fine Manipulation with fingers (right hand)						
Fine Manipulation with fingers (left hand)						
Operate foot pedals (right foot)						
Operate foot pedals (left foot)						

SAMPLE SUMMARY OF USING THE BODY FOR
NONEXERTIONAL ACTIVITIES

Although I am able to climb, stoop (bend), kneel, crouch, and crawl; I need frequent rest from such postures. I am able to balance at all times. (A person with a spinal cord injury or with cerebral palsy may not be able to take balancing for granted.) I am limited by my frequent need to change my body position. I am able to use both of my hands for handling, grasping, and fine finger dexterity. I would find power grasping or the grasping of a vibrating power tool tiring after a short time. I take a short rest break at least once per hour when I work on my computer keyboard. I find that I need a break after three or four hours of operating the foot pedals while driving my car on long trips.

**MY SUMMARY OF USING MY BODY FOR
NONEXERTIONAL ACTIVITIES**

_____

_____

_____

_____

_____

_____

_____

_____

_____

_____

_____

_____

_____

_____

_____

_____

_____

_____

_____

MY CURRENT EDUCATIONAL LEVELS

The Social Security Administration, Office of Hearings and Appeals has established educational categories to be used in disability determinations (1990, February, pp. 27-28). These categories have been used to make a chart for your use.

CATEGORIES	YES	NO

Illiteracy: The inability to read or write. Inability to read or write a simple message such as instructions or inventory lists, even though she is able to sign her name. Such persons usually have had little or no education.

Inability to Communicate in English: Because English is the dominant language of this country, a person who does not speak and understand English may find it difficult to perform or obtain a job regardless of the amount of education the person has in another language.

Marginal Education: Formal schooling at the 6th grade level or less is a marginal education. Abilities in reasoning, arithmetic, and language skills which allow performance of simple, unskilled types of jobs.

Limited Education: Formal schooling at the 7th grade through the 11th grade level. Abilities in reasoning, arithmetic, and language skills which do not allow performance of most of the more complex job duties needed in semiskilled or skilled jobs.

High School Education Plus: Includes the General Equivalency Diploma (GED). Ability in reasoning, arithmetic, and language skills which permits performance of semiskilled through skilled work.

Persons who have a high school education and beyond, and whose education is recent, are deemed able to enter semiskilled or skilled work without much difficulty. However, a person with a high school diploma or college degree which has not been used in the waged, skilled work world for 20 years or more, may not be able to enter waged, skilled work without additional education.

Date of my high school graduation or GED: _____

Date(s) of my college degree(s) or other education beyond high school: _____

MY CURRENT SKILL LEVELS

The Social Security Administration also defines Skills Levels according to the demands of the occupation. There are three categories defined as unskilled work, semiskilled work, and skilled work. Your completion of the chapter, *Analyzing, Respecting, and Celebrating Your Work*, means that you will be able to easily summarize your current skill development levels into these three broad categories by listing the categories of your achievement history into this chart. These categories are: 1) Saving My Own Life; 2) Childhood Achievements; 3) Adult Educational Achievements; 4) Adult Unwaged Work Achievements; 5) Adult Waged Work Achievements; and, 6) Miscellaneous.

Unskilled Work

(Requires no or little judgment to perform simple duties that you could learn on a new waged job or at home in unwaged work)

DATA

Comparing: I used this worker function in the following categories of *My Achievement History:*

Copying: I used this worker function in the following categories of *My Achievement History:*

PEOPLE

Taking Instructions-Helping: I used this worker function in the following categories of *My Achievement History:*

Serving: I used this worker function in the following categories of *My Achievement History:*

Speaking-Signaling: I used this worker function in the following categories of *My Achievement History:*

THINGS

Handling: I used this worker function in the following categories of My Achievement History:

Feeding-Offbearing: I used this worker function in the following categories of My Achievement History:

Tending: I used this worker function in the following categories of *My Achievement History:*

Semi-Skilled Work
(requires some skills but does not require performing the more complex work duties)

DATA

Computing: I used this worker function in the following categories of *My Achievement History:*

Compiling: I used this worker function in the following categories of *My Achievement History:*

PEOPLE

Persuading: I used this worker function in the following categories of *My Achievement History:*

Diverting: I used this worker function in the following categories of *My Achievement History:*

Supervising: I used this worker function in the following categories of **My Achievement History:**

THINGS

Manipulating: I used this worker function in the following categories of **My Achievement History:**

Driving-Operating: I used this worker function in the following categories of *My Achievement History:*

Operating-Controlling: I used this worker function in the following categories of *My Achievement History:*

Skilled Work
(Requires the performance of complex work duties)

DATA

Analyzing: I used this worker function in the following categories of *My Achievement History:*

Coordinating: I used this worker function in the following categories of *My Achievement History:*

Synthesizing: I used this worker function in the following categories of *My Achievement History:*

PEOPLE

Instructing: I used this worker function in the following categories of *My Achievement History:*

Negotiating: I used this worker function in the following categories of *My Achievement History:*

Mentoring: I used this worker function in the following categories of *My Achievement History:*

THINGS

Precision Working: I used this worker function in the following categories of *My Achievement History:*

Setting Up: I used this worker function in the following categories of *My Achievement History:*

My current skills levels are grouped primarily in Unskilled Work ?____

Semi-Skilled Work?_____   Skilled Work?_____

Now that you understand your vocational impairment issues/barriers; what are you going to do about it? The answer, of course, is to make a plan. Vocational impairments can be overcome, and you have taken most of the steps to do just that. You have faced *your* reality. You are now ready for moving on, moving through the flower.

> **TIP**
>
> You don't ever have to go it alone. This information is extremely valuable when working with a career and life planning counselor, vocational rehabilitation counselor or vocational expert, therapist, or employment assistance counselor.

section III. the plan – re-weaving your own life and work

*The importance of the Goddess in relation to the development of textiles can-
not be overemphasized. A variety of ancient myths and legends attribute the
invention of spinning and weaving to female deities, who are supposed to have
taught these skills to women and sanctified their work. The actual origins of
spinning are unknown, although evidence suggests that it was developed by
women sometime during the Paleolithic period, and in art, myth, and legend
spinning has been continuously portrayed as a female activity.*

Judy Chicago, 1980, p. 26

ten

introduction

Many ancient goddesses were described as the spinners of life *or* weavers of destiny, *characterizations that continued to be ascribed to female deities throughout the ages.*

Judy Chicago, 1980, p. 26

You are the spinner of your own life, the weaver of your own destiny, the teller of your own story (as in the modern meaning of spinning a yarn). Every exercise you have completed in this Workbook is part of your story. And what a story it has been! Tragedy, triumph, disaster, monsters, delays, setbacks, obstacles, lies, discoveries, hard truths, misunderstandings, legends, myths, lost heritage, death-defying feats, hair-raising escapes, and confrontations. In short, all the makings of a heroic quest, and a story worthy of the knights of the Round Table, *Indiana Jones and the Raiders of the Lost Ark* or the *Star Wars Trilogy*.

At this point, you may be looking over your shoulder for the hero. Who me? A hero? A heroic quest? Yes, because the recovery from abuse is women's quest plot. It is beyond "the old story of woman's destiny, the old marriage plot" (Heilbrun, 1988, p. 121). Recovery from abuse is the movement, the giving way "to another story for women, a quest plot" (Heilbrun, 1988, p. 121). When the search for the treasure is added to women's abuse recovery stories, then the quest plot for women becomes even more understandable, because all quest plots have treasures such as the Holy Grail, the Lost Ark, a lost heritage. The *treasure* for women is economic self-sufficiency, having your own money, having power and control over your own life, leaving behind any dependency you may have had on the old marriage plot to save you.

In the early days of the women's movement, I was asked to create and teach an introductory women's studies course for a community college. I asked the students to invite their significant others to a session for a general discussion of the then-startling and upsetting ideas emerging from the class. One woman brought her teen-age son. He listened intently to a discussion of why economic equality between women and men was not only fair, but necessary, and in the tradition of out-of-the-mouths-of-babes, raised his hand and asked, "But if women had as much money as men, why would they ever marry them?" He had, of course, put his young finger unerringly on the oppressive nature of the marriage plot for women. My reply was,

"Because they like them." There was a long silence while he and the rest of the class pondered this still-revolutionary notion. And why should there ever be any other reason for people to be together? Doesn't every person, regardless of gender, have the right to self-determination? To have the great adventure of her own life? To pursue her own quest? To spin her own yarn?

The purpose for this section of the Workbook is help you with your quest plot, to discover the means and methods for finding the treasure — the economic independence and self-sufficiency you deserve. This means that the old victim story has to go. Finding the treasure takes you beyond the survivor story too. Finding the treasure means that you are a hero, the hero of your own life (and perhaps, the hero of your children's lives as well).

> **TIP**
> You may find the word *hero* masculine, but some thinkers assign the word to Hera, the Leader of War and Queen of the Amazons in Antolia during the Bronze Age. From *A Feminist Dictionary* by Cheris Kramarae and Paula A. Treichler.

The next three chapters of the Workbook, *Making the Frame, Stretching the Self,* and *Weaving A Life,* emerge from the ancient tradition of the Goddess who sanctified the work of women, especially as they spun and wove; and from the modern tradition of the making of *The Dinner Party,* where women's needlework was also sanctified and revered. As a traumatic abuse survivor, you may not feel that you deserve the treasure, but remember that the work of your quest for the treasure is holy, sanctified, and emerges from an ancient and modern tradition. In this light, you will spin a web in *Making the Frame,* a method of writing and dreaming your ideal future into reality. In *Stretching the Self,* you will actualize your dream by discovering the possibilities, the resources which exist in your community. In *Weaving A Life,* you will learn how to sustain your vision in the face of those who would change it, try to tell your story, usurp your narrative, your yarn.

You will have moved from victim, to survivor, to hero. Blessed Be.

eleven

---

making the frame

*Usually, embroidery is done on a frame that allows the needleworker
to roll up the fabric and work on only one section at a time. But I
wanted the runners to be seen as paintings and the needleworkers to
deal with the overall picture plane as they worked.*

Judy Chicago, 1980, p. 16

In the making of *The Dinner Party*, Judy Chicago discovered that women do not
perceive the big picture because their work is often done in the corners, on the
edges, in cramped spaces — much in the way most embroidery is done, a small bit
at a time. This constricted way of doing our work affects our thinking, prevents us
from seeing the big picture. This constriction will be very familiar to abuse survivors since part of our abuse experience has been the distortion of our reality by our
perpetrators into their narrow view of what and who we are. Therefore it is very
important that in your career and life planning you open up your thinking to encompass the overall picture as the needleworkers did in the making of *The Dinner Party*.
In order to do this, large and adjustable frames were built out of hardwood so that
the frames could withstand the pressure of the needlework in a variety of positions
without twisting or distortion. Similarly, you will build an adjustable frame, and it
will stand up to the pressures of your life without twisting or distortion.

The first steps in constructing *your* frame is to dream, to think your ideal life.
Paula Gunn Allen's writing connects us back into the ancient female tradition of the
Goddess, the supreme being known as Spider Woman. Her name is translated as
Thought Woman or "Creating-through-Thinking Woman" (1989, p. 98). Leslie
Marmon Silko (1978, p. 1) describes a ceremony of cosmic significance which can
simultaneously heal a human, a stricken landscape, and a disorganized, discouraged
society. Her poem is a blessing, a ceremony, which illuminates the power of Spider
Woman.

Thought-woman, the spider
named things and
as she named them
they appeared.

She is sitting in her room
Thinking of a story now.
I'm telling you the story
she is thinking.

The power of the work you are about to do cannot be underestimated. When you do this work you evoke the power of Thought-Woman/Spider Woman. As *you name things, they will appear.* This is a case of what you ask for, you will get. In my first description of my ideal life, I wanted a video camera but my thoughts about video cameras were very outdated. I got a video camera given to me! I didn't even have to earn the money to buy one. The problem was that I had named the heavy, black and white cameras of the old days before the lightweight color cameras came into being! The point is, dream big, dream in detail, be specific.

Spider Woman's Dream – My Ideal Life

WHO? (*Who* do you want in your life? Your children? Maybe you want to have children, or maybe you want a new relationship with your children. Describe this new relationship. Do you want a life partner? Describe your ideal life partner. Maybe you want a new relationship with yourself and time alone to develop that relationship. Describe that. Who do you want in your waged work life? Do you want a boss? Or do you want to be the boss? Do you want to work by yourself, or with others, or in some combination of work alone and work with others? Describe this. Do you want to work with your peers or with people who have higher or lower educational and skill levels than you do? Describe this. Are these people your co-workers? Your clients? Your students? Do you want to work with groups or one on one? Perhaps some combination of this? What about age groups of people? Gender or race or ethnicity? Maybe you have a mission to work with African-American teenage girls or white adolescent boys. Write as much detail as you can.)

_____

_____

_____

_____

_____

_____

_____

_____

_____

_____

_____

Spider Woman's Dream – My Ideal Life continued...

WHAT? (The *what* of your ideal life refers to the things in your life. Do you want a house? What kind of a house? How big? What color? How many bedrooms? Is there an office? What about an art studio? A greenhouse? A garden? Stables? What's in your house? Artwork? Deep, soft couches? A swimming pool? Coffee grinder? Matching pots and pans? Do you have a car? A jet plane? What kind? What is in your workspace? A computer and printer? Be specific. A video camera (be very specific)? A drafting table? What are your tools? Do you have a set of Sears mechanic's tools? Which set? Are they in a toolbox on wheels? Paintbrushes? A set of gourmet chef kitchen knives? What does your workspace look like? Does it have a fireplace? Remember this is your *ideal* life. Bookshelves? Maybe it's a shop with woodworking tools? Does it have windows? Which way does it face? Do you get northern light? What about the floor? Carpet? Tile? A drain? What?)

_____

_____

_____

_____

_____

_____

_____

_____

_____

_____

_____

_____

Spider Woman's Dream – My Ideal Life continued...

WHEN? (*When* refers to the time elements of your life. How much time are you willing to commute to and from work? Maybe none? Maybe you work at home for wages? How much time are you willing to drive your children to all of their various activities? Maybe none. Maybe you live in a central location where your children walk to school and ballet lessons and soccer practice. Maybe you are willing to commute for hours at a time on an airplane as you fly to other cities or countries to do your waged work? Or maybe you are willing to drive an hour one way for waged work so that you can live in the country? How much time is spent in waged work in your ideal life? 80 hours per week? 20 hours per week? How much time do you spend with your children per week? Your lover? Your partner? By yourself? Engaged in hobbies or artmaking or sports? How do you spend your days? Your weekends? (It can be helpful to make a time line for your days which include the time you get up and a list of your activities hour by hour until you go to sleep.) How much vacation time do you need in a year in your ideal life? A month? A few days here and there?)

_____

_____

_____

_____

_____

_____

_____

_____

_____

_____

_____

_____

_____

_____

_____

_____

_____

_____

_____

_____

_____

_____

_____

_____

_____

_____

_____

_____

_____

Spider Woman's Dream – My Ideal Life continued...

WHERE? (*Where* refers to the geography of your ideal life. Do you live in the country, the wilderness, the city, the suburbs? Where is your waged work in relationship to your home life? Is your work national or international? Is your work in your home? Is there some combination of work in the home and out of the home? Do you grade papers at home, but teach at a school in the city? Do you have a country home and a city apartment? Where is your office, your studio, your business? In your ideal life, do you have a view of the city streets so you can watch people go by? Or perhaps you have a view of the treetops in the nearby national forest? Or maybe you work inside a photography studio developing photographs? Do you have the pleasures of a darkroom combined with the inspiration of your work on the ski slopes photographing skiers during the ski season? Maybe your work takes you to the rooftop gardens of large cities where you work as a landscaper in the sky? Where do you take your vacations? In London for the theater? In Yosemite for the hiking?)

_____

_____

_____

_____

_____

_____

_____

_____

_____

_____

_____

_____

_____

_____

_____

_____

_____

_____

_____

_____

_____

_____

_____

_____

_____

_____

_____

_____

_____

_____

Spider Woman's Dream – My Ideal Life continued...

WHY? (*Why* is the question of questions. Why refers to the purpose of *your* life. It is the *why am I here?* of your life. In a good life, you fulfill *your* purpose in life, not someone else's purpose or idea of what *your* life should be. This is the hero part of the yarn you are spinning, the story you are telling, the Spider Woman Dream you are dreaming. To live the purpose of *your* life is the life of a hero. It takes courage to live the life that is right for *you*. Curiously, Gloria Steinem and Maharishi Mahesh Yogi have the same thing to say on this point. The Maharishi advises that it is possible to live another person's *dharma* but it is not good for *your* evolution. *Dharma* is a Hindu term which refers to one's duty, purpose, or mission in life. (Don't confuse this term with *karma* which refers to the principal that for every action there is an equal and opposite reaction.) There is no English equivalent for the word *dharma*, but it is a useful word because it contains meanings which includes one's work in life, one's purpose in relating to others in family and work, and the spiritual meaning of one's purpose in life. The Maharishi's advice is restated by Gloria Steinem when she says that instead of doing it, women marry it. That is, women confuse themselves when they think they cannot dream big or do what they want to do, and so they take the conventional way out—they marry a man who does what they want to do. The Maharishi points out that this is not good for our development and evolution as human beings. Chances are someone else will never live the life we want the way we would if only we had the courage to live it ourselves. Naming the *dharma,* or purpose, or why of your life is an act of self liberation. It is the center of Spider Woman's web. It is the lynchpin which holds the frame of your life together. In the early days of my recovery, I carried my written purpose of my life in my appointment book. Whenever I felt overwhelmed and confused, I opened my appointment book and read it. It was and is the answer to my questions of questions, *Why am I here?* "Oh yes," I could tell myself. "The purpose of my life is to express the experience of my life through writing, teaching, and healing." *Your* purpose can probably be stated in one sentence as well. The breathing exercise described in *Overcoming Verbal-Emotional Abuse* is useful in hearing *your* answer to this question. The guided meditation in the same chapter may also help. You may choose to ask your guide for the answer to your question.)

The purpose of my life is to:

_____

_____

_____

_____

_____

Now that you have identified the purpose of your life, you are ready to do some management by objective or *MBO* as it is called at the Harvard Business School. Every plan, every organization, every project has or should have a mission statement. The purpose of your life is your mission statement for your career and life plan. The next steps are to identify goals which fit under *your* mission statement, and the objectives or the means by which you will fulfill *your* goals.

TIP

If you find yourself vacillating wildly between *I'm-the-worst-person-in-the-world-lower-than-a-worm* and *I-want-to-be-a-billionaire-in-two-weeks-because-the-world-owes-me*, regard this as a vanity of the victim attack, and shrug it off. One of the effects of traumatic abuse is going to the extremes of self-loathing or self-aggrandizment, or *the-nobody-has-suffered-as-much-as-I-have-and-therefore-I-deserve-to-win-the-lottery* syndrome. As abuse survivors, we don't have much experience in walking the middle way, the path of moderation. The identification of objectives or means to fulfill our goals has a tendency to bring us down to earth with a thump because we are forced to face the step by step work it takes to make our dreams come true. A suggested affirmation is, *I, (name) enjoy every aspect of the work of fulfilling my purpose and goals in life.*

TIP

Most people have only three or four goals. Objectives or the means by which these broadly based goals are to be fulfilled are the specific detailed lists. Goals and objectives change over time, but one's life purpose usually stays the same.

The Management by Objective Career and Life Plan Statement is based in time. That is, goals and objectives are set inside a time frame. I recommend that this time frame be in ten year segments because our thinking is then expanded beyond the usual abuse survivor constrictions, including the posttraumatic stress disorder symptom: *I'm not going to live very long, or I could die at any moment, so why plan?* The very act of writing down your ideal life, your life purpose, your goals and objectives, and a timeline releases your energy so that the actualizing of your dreams becomes possible, so that the Spider Woman/Thought Woman power within us comes alive, and gives us the bridge over the posttraumatic stress disorder symptoms which may be with us still.

I have placed the Ten-Year Plan charts next to the Management by Objective Career and Life Plan Statements because it will be easier for you to work that way. However, it is important to read the Using the Worklife Expectancy and Life Expectancy Tables in Thinking About Your Ten-Year Plan Timeline section in this chapter *before* you complete your ten-year plan.

A Sample Management By Objective Career and Life Statement for a 33-year-old Woman.

My purpose in life is to work with children in my home and on the job.

GOAL #1 – To complete my education:
  a) by completing my A.A. degree at my community college.
  b) by transferring to the nearby state university to obtain my bachelor's degree and elementary school teaching credential.
  c) by applying for scholarships and financial aid in order to finance my education.
  d) by applying for a child care grant and work study money in order to finance my education.
  e) by using the services of the women's center and the disabled students services center at the colleges I attend.
  f) by applying for jobs in child day care centers, or as a teacher's aide as soon as I have completed coursework in preschool and elementary school education.

GOAL #2 – To improve my parenting skills with my three children:
  a) by taking parenting skills classes and seminars at my community college.
  b) by using the crisis line when I feel out of control with my children.
  c) by continuing in my support group offered by the battered women's agency in my community.
  d) by asking for help when I need it.
  e) by arranging child care exchanges with mothers I trust so that I can take a break.

GOAL #3 – To maintain good mental and physical health by meeting the following *objectives:*
  a) by telling the truth.
  b) by actively maintaining and nurturing healthy and loving relationships in my life with family, friends, colleagues, and coworkers.
  c) by asserting myself appropriately, especially in the face of verbal-emotional abuse.
  d) by maintaining my regular exercise program of daily walking.
  e) by maintaining balance in my life between work and play.
  f) by maintaining and improving my positive health habits such as good food, proper rest, regular pap smears.
  g) by getting abuse recovery therapy.
  h) by locating a 12-Step Group I like for my substance abuse issues.

GOAL #4 – To move toward financial self-sufficiency:

   a) by understanding that living on AFDC is a temporary situation.

   b) by being willing to participate in the work/training programs under AFDC, but not allowing the AFDC people to define my goals for me.

   c) by working with a credit counselor in order to reorganize my debts and to understand which of these debts are mine and which are my husband's.

   d) by working with legal aide to get a no cost or low cost divorce so that I have no more responsibility for my husband's debts, and to get child support money.

A Sample 10-year Plan 1994 to 2004 – Age 33 to 43 Years

Year	Goal 1	Goal 2	Goal 3	Goal 4
1994	Apply for scholarships and financial aide. Child care grant. Apply for school.	Take parenting class. Call crisis line. Go to support group.	Find therapist (free or low cost). Find 12-step group. Get pap smear.	Check out AFDC work programs and educational opportunities. Go to credit counselor. Go to legal aide.
1995	Take at least 1/2 time course load. Apply for work study.	Take parenting class. Go to support group.	Work with therapist. 12-Step. Pap Smear.	Finish up divorce. Get regular child support through district attorney.
1996	Get to full-time course load.	Take parenting class.	12-Step. Pap smear.	Make plan for getting off AFDC by 1997.
1997	Get A.A. degree in early childhood education.	Practice. Practice. Practice.	12-Step. Pap smear.	Get job as child care worker and get off AFDC.
1998	Take a summer break. Apply for state university.	Practice. Practice. Practice.	12-Step. Get pap smear.	Work as child care worker. Use food stamps and housing grant only.
1999	Start B.A. degree at university in Fall '98 or Spring '99. Apply for loans and aide.	Practice. Practice. Practice.	Get pap smear. 12-Step.	Work study at university or child care worker at university.
2000	Continue B.A. full-time.	Practice. Practice.	Get pap smear. 12-Step.	Work.
2001	Continue B.A. Graduate and apply for grad school.	Practice. Practice.	12-Step. Pap smear.	Work.
2002	Get loan or grant for teaching credential study, apply for jobs.	Practice. Practice.	12-Step. Pap smear.	No work, full-time teaching internship.
2003	Get job as school teacher.	Kids all off to work or college.	12-Step. Pap smear.	Elementary school teacher.
2004	School teacher. Apply for master's degree in teaching.	Kids home for visits only.	12-Step. Pap smear.	Figure out how to buy housing, stop renting, pay off school debts.

All other objectives are continuous over the ten years such as asking for help, telling the truth, maintaining healthy relationships.

TIP

In the year 2004, this woman may wish to create a new career and life plan and place it inside the ten years between ages 43 to 53.

**A Sample Management By Objective Career and Life Statement
for a 54-year-old Woman**

My purpose in life is to serve the needs of women and children by changing the laws.

GOAL #1 – To become an attorney-at-law:
- a) by completing my application for law schools in my area.
- b) by studying for the LSAT examination and taking it.
- c) by entering law school.
- d) by considering going to law school at night if I cannot get a scholarship.
- e) by passing the state bar examination.
- f) by entering the practice of law.

GOAL #2 – To complete my recovery from years of domestic violence:
- a) by continuing my volunteer work at the shelter.
- b) by completing my volunteer advocacy training in writing restraining orders for formerly battered women.
- c) by attending my support group on a regular basis.
- d) by doing my affirmation work on a regular basis.
- e) by doing my exercise program as prescribed by the physical therapist.
- f) by knowing that I can be an attorney myself, instead of marrying an attorney.
- g) by working with a therapist on my issues of sexual dysfunction.

GOAL #3 – To establish my economic independence:
- a) by completing a vocational plan to present to the judge in divorce court which will provide me with spousal support and law school tuition for at least four years.
- b) by applying for part-time staff jobs at the domestic violence shelter where I now volunteer, or by applying for part-time jobs in law firms (clerical or legal assistant).
- c) by making sure that my young adult children are provided with college education money when the divorce settlement is reached.
- d) by working with a financial advisor to determine how to sell the house and set up a retirement plan for myself.
- e) by taking community college classes and workshops in financial planning and money management.
- f) by applying for my own credit cards and getting everything into my own name.

The objectives such as *the physical therapy exercises, affirmation work, and knowing she can be an attorney instead of marrying one (probably an affirmation)* are presumed to be continuous over the ten-year period.

A Sample 10-year Plan 1994 to 2004 – Age 54 to 64 Years

Year	Goal 1	Goal 2	Goal 3
1994	Complete application process. Study for LSAT exam. Take LSAT and start law school.	Volunteer work. Learn to write restraining orders. Support group.	Complete vocational plan for judge to get spousal support and tuition for law school for four years. Get credit cards and records in my name.
1995	Law school.	Volunteer advocate for battered women in the courtroom. Find rapist.	Use spousal support wisely. Monitor child support for college.
1996	Finish law school. Study for bar exam.	Volunteer advocate in courtroom. Work with therapist.	Use spousal support. Monitor child support.
1997	Pass bar exam. Apply for jobs. Get job as attorney.	Volunteer advocate in courtroom. Find new support group.	Work as legal assistant or work as staff for domestic violence shelter. Make transition off spousal support. Monitor child support.
1998	Work as attorney.	Pro bono work for battered women.	Sell the house and set up retirement plan. Take classes and seminars in financial planning. Buy smaller house/condo.
1999	Work as an attorney.	Pro bono work for battered women.	Work with financial adviser.
2000	Work as an attorney.	Pro bono work for battered women. Take a vacation.	Learn how to invest in socially responsible companies.
2001	Work as an attorney. Get legal specialist certification in family law.	Pro bono work for battered women.	Maintain financial independence.
2002	Work as an attorney. Hold office in professional organizations.	Train legal advocates for battered women.	Maintain financial health.
2003	Work as an attorney. Work on state and federal legislation to change laws on the behalf of battered women and their children.	Train legal advocates for battered women.	Maintain financial health.
2004	Work as an attorney. Continue work on legislation.	Take a vacation.	Maintain financial health.

TIP
Women who are 64 should also make a ten-year plan for the years between 64 and 74.

My Management By Objective Career and Life Plan Statement

My purpose in life is to:

_____

GOAL #1 – I will fulfill this goal by meeting the following *objectives:*

a) _____

b) _____

c) _____

d) _____

e) _____

GOAL #2 – I will fulfill this goal by meeting the following *objectives:*

a) _____

b) _____

c) _____

d) _____

e) _____

GOAL #3 – I will fulfill this goal by meeting the following *objectives:*

a) _____

b) _____

c) _____

d) _____

e) _____

GOAL #4 – I will fulfill this goal by meeting the following *objectives:*

a) _____

b) _____

c) _____

d) _____

e) _____

My Ten-year Plan 199__ to 200__ – Age _____ to _____ Years

Year	Goal 1	Goal 2	Goal 3	Goal 4
199__				
199__				
199__				
199__				
199__				
200__				
200__				
200__				
200__				
200__				
200__				

Using Worklife Expectancy and Life Expectancy Tables in Thinking About Your Ten-year Plan Timeline

Age, race, and gender all influence how long we live and how long we are active in the waged work world. The United States Department of Health and Human Services, Public Health Service, National Center for Health Statistics published *Table A-2. Life and Worklife Expectancies for Men by Race, 1979-1980* (see Figure 1) and *Table A-5, Life and Worklife Expectancies for Women by Race, 1979-1980* (see Figure 2). No statistical data can accurately predict the life span or the worklife expectancy of any one individual. These statistics are generalizations, and include information from thousands, even millions of people. However, we can get a general idea of how long we can expect to live and to work in the waged work world.

The tables are easy to use. For example, let's compare what happens to a 33-year-old person by gender and race. Using Table A-2, go to the column titled, *Age* and find 33. Moving to the right, we find a column titled, *Life Expectancy* which is under another heading, *White Men*. A 33-year-old white man has 40.5 years of life expectancy remaining, or his expected death is at 73.5 years. Moving to the right again, the column under the heading, *Expectation of Active Life by Labor Force Status,* with the column titled, *Total* under that, we discover that our 33-year-old white man can expect to have 26.8 active years in the waged labor market, or that he will work until he is 59.8 years of age. If our 33-year-old person is African-American or other (the government does not keep statistics by all minority groups which makes all of us either white, Black, or other statistically), and male, then we find that his life expectancy is 36.4 years or 4.1 years less than his white brother. His worklife expectancy is 4.5 years less than his white brother.

Moving to Table A-5, we find that a 33-year-old white woman has a life expectancy of 47.0 years or can expect to die at age 80 as compared to a 43.5 years of life expectancy for an African-American woman with an expected death at age 76.5. The white woman can expect to live 3.5 years longer than her Black sister. Their worklife expectancies are closer together, however. The 33-year-old white woman can expect to work 19 years and the Black woman 18.3 years.

As we can now see, women live longer than men, but their waged work lives are shorter. The 33-year-old white man and white woman have a difference of 7.8 years of waged worklife expectancies, and the 33-year-old Black man and Black woman have a gap of four years.

What accounts for the differences between women and men and their expected years in the waged work world? Researchers have frequently noted that women's participation in the waged labor market is discontinuous. That is, women drop in and out of the labor market to stay in the home to care for children or other family members. Men still do not have the primary responsibility for these necessary unwaged work duties. Other researchers indicate that women face age discrimination in the labor market sooner than men, and this also shortens women's waged worklife expectancies.

What this means is that you may find yourself facing old age in poverty because a shorter waged worklife means less money earned, less money saved for retirement, less opportunity to create and contribute to a pension plan. Combine these dismal facts with the earnings by women which are significantly less than that of male earnings, we find that our 33-year-old white woman will have a 28-year life span in her older years when she is not working for wages, but will somehow have to eat, house herself, provide for medical care, and other living expenses. Her African-American sister faces 23.2 years of trying to manage, and she faces inequality in wages not only because she is a woman, but because she is Black. Her average wages are lower than that of every other group mentioned here.

TIP

Breathe! Right about now, all your bag lady fears are probably circling about in your brain like vultures. Read on, there is hope. Remember Judy Chicago's words, "growth takes places by starting where we really are."

Table A-2. Life and Worklife Expectancies for Men by Race. 1979-80.
(Average years remaining)

	White men				Black and other men			
Age	Life Expectancy*	Expectation of active life by labor force status			Life Expectancy*	Expectation of active life by labor force status		
		Total	Currently Active	Currently inactive		Total	Currently Active	Currently inactive
x	$\dot{e}\dot{}_x$	$\dot{e}^a_x$	$^a e^a_x$	$^i e^a_x$	$\dot{e}\dot{}_x$	$\dot{e}^a_x$	$^a e^a_x$	$^i e^a_x$
	(1)	(2)	(3)	(4)	(5)	(6)	(7)	(8)
16	56.1	39.9	40.6	39.1	51.4	33.6	34.3	33.2
17	55.2	39.4	40.0	38.4	50.4	33.2	33.9	32.7
18	54.3	38.8	39.4	37.8	49.5	32.8	33.5	32.2
19	53.3	38.2	38.8	37.1	48.6	32.4	33.0	31.7
20	52.4	37.5	38.1	36.4	47.6	31.9	32.4	31.1
21	51.5	36.9	37.4	35.6	46.8	31.3	31.8	30.4
22	50.6	36.1	36.6	34.9	45.9	30.7	31.1	29.7
23	49.7	35.4	35.8	34.1	45.0	30.0	30.4	29.0
24	48.8	34.6	35.0	33.2	44.1	29.3	29.7	28.3
25	47.9	33.8	34.2	32.4	43.3	28.6	28.9	27.5
26	47.0	32.9	33.3	31.5	42.4	27.9	28.2	26.6
27	46.1	32.1	32.4	30.6	41.5	27.1	27.4	25.8
28	45.2	31.2	31.6	29.7	40.7	26.4	26.6	25.0
29	44.2	30.3	30.7	28.7	39.8	25.6	25.8	24.1
30	43.3	29.5	29.8	27.7	39.0	24.8	25.0	23.2
31	42.4	28.6	28.9	26.7	38.1	24.0	24.2	22.3
32	41.4	27.7	28.0	25.7	37.2	23.2	23.4	21.3
33	40.5	26.8	27.1	24.7	36.4	22.3	22.7	20.3
34	39.6	25.9	26.2	23.7	35.5	21.5	21.9	19.3
35	38.6	25.0	25.3	22.7	34.7	20.7	21.1	18.2
36	37.7	24.1	24.4	21.7	33.8	19.9	20.4	17.1
37	36.8	23.2	23.5	20.7	33.0	19.1	19.6	16.0
38	35.9	22.3	22.6	19.6	32.2	18.4	18.9	15.0
39	34.9	21.4	21.7	18.6	31.3	17.6	18.1	14.2
40	34.0	20.5	20.9	17.5	30.5	16.8	17.4	13.4
41	33.1	19.6	20.0	16.4	29.7	16.0	16.7	12.6
42	32.2	18.7	19.1	15.4	28.9	15.3	16.0	11.9
43	31.3	17.8	18.3	14.3	28.1	14.5	15.2	11.1
44	30.4	16.9	17.4	13.2	27.3	13.8	14.5	10.4
45	29.5	16.1	16.6	12.1	26.5	13.1	13.8	9.7
46	28.6	15.2	15.8	11.2	25.8	12.4	13.1	8.9
47	27.8	14.4	14.9	10.3	25.0	11.6	12.4	8.1
48	26.9	13.5	14.1	9.4	24.3	10.9	11.7	7.3
49	26.1	12.7	13.4	8.6	23.5	10.2	11.0	6.5
50	25.2	11.9	12.6	7.8	22.8	9.5	10.4	5.7
51	24.4	11.1	11.8	7.1	22.1	8.8	9.7	4.9
52	23.6	10.3	11.1	6.3	21.5	8.1	9.1	4.3
53	22.8	9.5	10.3	5.6	20.8	7.4	8.4	3.7
54	22.0	8.7	9.6	5.0	20.2	6.8	7.8	3.2
55	21.3	8.0	8.9	4.4	19.5	6.1	7.2	2.8
56	20.5	7.2	8.2	3.8	18.9	5.5	6.6	2.5
57	19.7	6.5	7.5	3.3	18.3	4.9	6.0	2.2
58	19.0	5.8	6.9	2.9	17.7	4.3	5.6	1.9
59	18.3	5.2	6.3	2.5	17.1	3.7	5.1	1.8
60	17.6	4.5	5.8	2.2	16.5	3.3	4.7	1.6
61	16.9	4.0	5.4	2.0	15.9	2.9	4.4	1.5
62	16.2	3.5	5.0	1.8	15.4	2.5	4.1	1.4
63	15.6	3.1	4.7	1.5	14.9	2.2	3.8	1.3
64	14.9	2.7	4.4	1.3	14.3	2.0	3.6	1.2
65	14.3	2.3	4.2	1.2	13.8	1.8	3.5	1.1
66	13.7	2.1	4.0	1.0	13.3	1.6	3.4	1.0
67	13.1	1.8	3.8	.8	12.8	1.4	3.3	.9
68	12.5	1.6	3.6	.7	12.3	1.3	3.2	.7
69	11.9	1.4	3.5	.5	11.8	1.2	3.0	.6
70	11.4	1.2	3.3	.4	11.4	1.0	2.9	.4
71	10.9	1.1	3.1	.3	10.9	.9	2.7	.3
72	10.4	.9	2.9	.2	10.5	.7	2.6	.2
73	9.9	.8	2.6	.1	10.0	.6	2.3	.1
74	9.4	.7	2.3	.1	9.6	.5	1.8	.0
75	8.9	.6	1.8	.0	9.2	.3	1.3	.0

* Mortality rates used reflect racial differentials in survival.

Figure 1

Table A-5. Life and Worklife Expectancies for Women by Race. 1979-80.

(Average years remaining)

Age	White women				Black and other women			
	Life Expectancy*	Expectation of active life by labor force status			Life Expectancy*	Expectation of active life by labor force status		
		Total	Currently Active	Currently inactive		Total	Currently Active	Currently inactive
x	$\overset{\cdot}{e}_x$	$\overset{\cdot}{e}{}^a_x$	$\overset{a}{e}{}^a_x$	$\overset{i}{e}{}^a_x$	$\overset{\cdot}{e}_x$	$\overset{\cdot}{e}{}^a_x$	$\overset{a}{e}{}^a_x$	$\overset{i}{e}{}^a_x$
	(1)	(2)	(3)	(4)	(5)	(6)	(7)	(8)
16	63.4	29.6	30.3	28.9	59.7	27.8	28.6	27.3
17	62.5	29.1	29.8	28.2	58.7	27.5	28.4	26.9
18	61.5	28.5	29.2	27.6	57.7	27.1	28.0	26.5
19	60.5	27.9	28.6	27.0	56.8	26.7	27.5	26.1
20	59.6	27.3	28.0	26.3	55.8	26.3	27.1	25.5
21	58.6	26.7	27.4	25.5	54.8	25.8	26.6	25.0
22	57.6	26.0	26.7	24.8	53.9	25.3	26.1	24.3
23	56.7	25.4	26.1	24.1	52.9	24.7	25.5	23.7
24	55.7	24.7	25.5	23.3	52.0	24.2	24.9	23.0
25	54.7	24.1	24.9	22.6	51.0	23.5	24.3	22.3
26	53.8	23.4	24.2	21.9	50.1	22.9	23.7	21.6
27	52.8	22.8	23.6	21.2	49.2	22.3	23.1	20.9
28	51.8	22.1	23.0	20.6	48.2	21.6	22.5	20.2
29	50.9	21.5	22.4	19.9	47.3	21.0	21.8	19.4
30	49.9	20.8	21.8	19.2	46.3	20.3	21.2	18.7
31	48.9	20.2	21.2	18.6	45.4	19.7	20.5	17.9
32	48.0	19.6	20.6	17.9	44.5	19.0	19.9	17.2
33	47.0	19.0	20.0	17.2	43.5	18.3	19.3	16.5
34	46.0	18.3	19.4	16.6	42.6	17.7	18.6	15.7
35	45.1	17.7	18.7	15.9	41.7	17.0	18.0	15.0
36	44.1	17.0	18.1	15.2	40.7	16.3	17.4	14.2
37	43.1	16.4	17.5	14.4	39.8	15.7	16.8	13.5
38	42.2	15.8	16.9	13.7	38.9	15.0	16.2	12.8
39	41.2	15.1	16.2	12.9	38.0	14.4	15.6	12.1
40	40.3	14.4	15.6	12.2	37.1	13.8	15.0	11.4
41	39.3	13.8	15.0	11.4	36.2	13.1	14.5	10.7
42	38.4	13.1	14.3	10.6	35.3	12.5	13.9	10.1
43	37.5	12.4	13.7	9.9	34.5	11.9	13.4	9.5
44	36.5	11.8	13.1	9.2	33.6	11.3	12.8	8.9
45	35.6	11.1	12.5	8.4	32.7	10.8	12.3	8.3
46	34.7	10.5	12.0	7.8	31.9	10.2	11.7	7.7
47	33.8	9.9	11.4	7.1	31.1	9.6	11.2	7.1
48	32.9	9.2	10.9	6.5	30.2	9.0	10.6	6.6
49	32.0	8.6	10.3	5.9	29.4	8.5	10.1	6.0
50	31.1	8.0	9.8	5.3	28.6	7.9	9.5	5.5
51	30.2	7.4	9.3	4.7	27.8	7.4	9.0	4.9
52	29.3	6.9	8.8	4.2	27.0	6.8	8.5	4.4
53	28.4	6.3	8.3	3.7	26.2	6.3	8.0	3.9
54	27.6	5.8	7.8	3.3	25.5	5.7	7.5	3.5
55	26.7	5.3	7.3	2.9	24.7	5.2	7.0	3.0
56	25.9	4.7	6.8	2.5	23.9	4.7	6.5	2.7
57	25.0	4.3	6.3	2.2	23.2	4.2	6.1	2.3
58	24.2	3.8	5.9	1.9	22.4	3.8	5.6	2.0
59	23.4	3.4	5.4	1.7	21.7	3.4	5.2	1.8
60	22.6	3.0	5.1	1.5	21.0	3.0	4.8	1.5
61	21.8	2.6	4.7	1.3	20.3	2.6	4.5	1.3
62	21.0	2.3	4.4	1.2	19.6	2.3	4.2	1.1
63	20.2	2.0	4.2	1.0	19.0	2.0	3.9	1.0
64	19.4	1.8	4.0	.9	18.3	1.7	3.7	.8
65	18.7	1.5	3.8	.8	17.7	1.5	3.4	.7
66	17.9	1.4	3.6	.6	17.0	1.3	3.2	.6
67	17.2	1.2	3.5	.5	16.4	1.1	3.0	.5
68	16.4	1.0	3.3	.5	15.7	.9	2.9	.4
69	15.7	.9	3.2	.4	15.1	.8	2.8	.3
70	15.0	.8	3.0	.3	14.5	.7	2.7	.2
71	14.3	.7	2.8	.2	13.9	.6	2.6	.2
72	13.6	.6	2.6	.2	13.4	.5	2.6	.1
73	13.0	.5	2.3	.1	12.9	.5	2.3	.1
74	12.3	.4	1.9	.0	12.3	.4	1.9	.0
75	11.7	.3	1.3	.0	11.8	.4	1.4	.0

* Mortality rates used reflect racial differentials in survival.

Figure 2

My Current Life Expectancy, Worklife Expectancy, and Retirement Years Expectancy

You can locate your life expectancy and worklife expectancy by using the tables as I did for the 33-year-old person. Simply locate your age under Table A-5 and move to the section in the table which most accurately reflects your racial status.

My current life expectancy is _____ years.

My current worklife expectancy is _____ years.

I currently have an expected _____ years of "retirement" to plan for, to avoid living in poverty. (Subtract your worklife expectancy from your life expectancy.)

Changing Your Worklife Expectancy

Although we do not have the power to change our sex, race, or age, we do have the power to change our statistical worklife expectancy. The most important factor in prolonging our worklife expectancy, and in increasing our overall lifetime earnings (and retirement savings and pension plan contributions) is education. Vocational experts refer to this as the *age earning cycle*. The more education a person has, the longer they remain in the labor market and the longer their earnings remain at higher levels, instead of declining when age discrimination takes its toll.

Table 8, Average Earnings By Education, Females, 1986 (Figure 3) was published by the United States Department of Labor, Bureau of Labor Statistics. No distinctions are made by race in this table. Inflation would probably make the wages listed on this 1986 table higher today, but it is the effect of education on wages that we are examining here, and this table will, hopefully, shock you into an understanding of the value of education. Our 33-year-old every woman on this table can expect to have average annual earnings of $9,575 with an 8th grade educational level. Her peak earnings at age 52 years are $11,829, and then the decline sets in until her earnings at age 69 years return close to her earnings of 33 years at $9,086. This presumes she had been able to work to age 69 years for a total of 36 years in the labor market. As we know, this is unlikely because her projected overall worklife expectancy overall was only 19 years as a white woman and 18.3 years if she were a Black woman.

Even one to three years of high school improves things dramatically, since our 33-year-old every woman now has $12,418 average annual earnings. If she had graduated from high school, her earnings jump to $15,832 annually, and with one to three years of college, jump again to $19,413. College graduation improves the average earnings to $23,801, and beyond that (advanced degrees) to $29,658. The message is, education pays off.

Table 8
Average Annual Earnings By Education, Females
1986
Education Level

Age	<8	8	1-3 hs	4 hs	1-3 col	4 col	5+ col
18	10,982	9,620	9,361	10,224	---------	---------	---------
19	10,991	9,617	9,633	10,627	---------	---------	---------
20	11,000	9,614	9,914	11,045	11,917	---------	---------
21	11,009	9,611	10,202	11,480	12,547	---------	---------
22	11,018	9,608	10,499	11,933	13,209	18,771	---------
23	11,027	9,605	10,804	12,403	13,907	19,318	---------
24	11,035	9,602	11,118	12,891	14,641	19,881	20,318
25	11,044	9,599	11,442	13,399	15,414	20,461	21,278
26	11,053	9,596	11,775	13,927	16,228	21,057	22,284
27	11,062	9,593	12,117	14,475	17,085	21,671	23,337
28	11,071	9,590	12,172	14,721	17,504	22,042	24,440
29	11,080	9,587	11,228	14,972	17,933	22,419	25,595
30	11,090	9,584	12,283	15,226	18,373	22,803	26,804
31	11,099	9,581	12,339	15,485	18,824	23,194	28,071
32	11,108	9,578	12,395	15,748	19,286	23,592	29,398
33	11,117	9,575	12,418	15,832	19,413	23,801	29,658
34	11,126	9,572	12,441	15,916	19,541	24,012	29,921
35	11,135	9,569	12,463	16,001	19,670	24,225	30,186
36	11,144	9,566	12,486	16,086	19,800	24,440	30,453
37	11,153	9,563	12,508	16,171	19,931	24,657	30,724
38	11,162	9,561	12,519	16,359	19,908	24,829	30,350
39	11,171	9,558	12,531	16,549	19,886	25,002	29,981
40	11,180	9,555	12,542	16,741	19,864	25,177	29,616
41	11,001	9,763	12,554	16,936	19,842	25,353	29,255
42	10,825	9,075	12,565	17,133	19,820	25,529	28,899
43	10,651	10,192	12,598	17,012	19,709	25,053	29,289
44	10,481	10,414	12,630	16,892	19,598	24,586	29,684
45	10,313	10,641	12,663	16,773	19,488	24,127	30,085
46	10,148	10,873	12,696	16,655	19,378	23,677	30,491
47	9,985	11,109	12,729	16,538	19,269	23,235	30,902
48	9,825	11,351	12,932	16,627	19,386	23,762	30,210
49	9,668	11,598	13,139	16,716	19,504	24,301	29,534
50	9,513	11,851	13,348	16,805	19,622	24,853	28,873
51	9,705	11,840	13,561	16,895	19,741	25,417	28,227
52	9,902	11,829	13,777	16,986	19,860	25,993	27,596
53	10,103	11,819	13,788	16,877	19,588	25,661	27,839
54	10,307	11,808	13,798	16,769	19,310	25,443	28,084
55	10,516	11,797	13,809	16,662	19,053	25,008	28,331
56	10,729	11,787	13,820	16,555	18,792	24,688	28,580
57	10,946	11,776	13,830	16,449	18,534	24,372	28,832
58	10,486	11,766	13,350	16,421	18,424	23,295	28,202
59	10,046	11,755	12,887	16,393	18,314	22,266	27,585
60	9,624	11,744	12,439	16,366	18,205	21,282	26,982
61	9,219	11,414	12,007	16,338	18,097	20,342	26,392
62	8,832	11,093	11,590	16,310	17,989	19,443	25,815
63	8,461	10,782	11,188	15,753	17,882	19,584	25,251
64	8,106	10,479	10,800	15,216	17,775	17,763	24,699
65	7,765	10,184	10,425	14,696	17,670	16,978	24,159
66	7,439	9,898	10,063	14,195	17,565	16,228	23,631
67	7,126	9,620	9,713	13,710	17,460	15,511	23,114
68	6,827	9,349	9,376	13,242	17,356	14,826	22,609
69	6,540	9,086	9,051	12,354	17,253	14,171	22,115

Figure 3

My Current Life Expectancy, Worklife Expectancy, and Retirement Years Expectancy

---

My current age is _____.

My current educational level is: _____

My projected average annual earnings now (according to Table 8) are:

My peak earnings take place at age _____years in the amount of_____.

My projected average annual earnings at age 69 years are:_____.

My current worklife expectancy is _____years.

I have _____years of "retirement" to plan for now (if I do nothing to change my worklife expectancy).

There are at least two reasons for investing your time, yourself, and your money into education. The first is obviously financial, and the second has to do with your purpose in life. The most fortunate women can combine these two reasons as the 33 year-old woman can do in the Sample Management by Objective Career & Life Plan Statement for a 33-year-old Woman. As we know, her worklife expectancy is 19 years even if she does nothing to increase her educational level. This means that even if it takes her eight or nine years to complete her degree and credential, she will have 10 to 11 years (and probably more) to increase her earnings, extend her worklife expectancy, and increase her chances for more prosperous retirement years. Simultaneously, she will be fulfilling her life purpose. Therefore, her proposed educational effort is a good investment.

The 54-year-old woman has only 5.8 years of worklife expectancy if she is white, and only 5.7 years of worklife expectancy remaining if she is Black. On the other hand, she faces 27.6 years of life expectancy or at least 21.8 retirement years to plan for as a white woman, or 19.8 years of retirement if as a Black woman. Why would a 54-year-old woman go to law school as indicated in the Sample Management by Objective for a 54-year-old Woman? She may be able to extend her worklife expectancy, and this will be very helpful in getting a higher level of Social Security income upon retirement. This is true even if she manages to be in the waged work world for ten years or less after law school. She may be able to save some money for her retirement years during that time, but the most important reason may not be financial. It may be that this is the only opportunity she has had to fulfill her purpose in life.

We don't just work for money. (Women sure don't. If women worked only for money, the world structure as we now know it would collapse.) Work has what vocational experts term *hedonic value*. That is, the pleasures of work. We work to be of service to others. We work to have the pleasure of using our brains, our hands, our hearts. We work for status and power. We work to bring about change, or for the sheer pleasure of being creative. We work to feel good about ourselves as productive members of society.

Therefore when you are working on your career and life plan statement goals and objectives, and placing them inside the ten-year plan timeline, don't ignore either the importance of money in your life, or the importance of pleasure in your work. You deserve both prosperity and pleasure.

Now return to your Management by Objective Career & Life Plan Statement, and complete your ten-year timeline.

In the next chapter, *Stretching the Self*, we will explore the use of resources available to you in making your Spider Woman/Thought Woman dreams come true.

twelve

---

stretching the self

The whole idea of artmaking as an involvement with materials, process, forms or "craft" was entirely foreign to me. When, in sculpture class, the teacher had given lectures on long, elaborate, technical processes, I had barely been able to contain my boredom. My male friends, although as bored as I was, took voluminous notes—preparations, I later discovered, for the time when they would get jobs teaching sculpture and setting up sculpture shops. No one had ever suggested to me that I would have to "make a living," so I was not involved in "preparing" myself for a job. (I supposed I just assumed that "somehow I would get along.")

Judy Chicago, 1979, pp. 31-32

Sounds like a song, doesn't it? *Somehow I'll just get along, and someday my prince will come.* Both scenarios are unlikely in this day and age where women are nearly 50 percent of the waged labor market, and more than half of marriages end in divorce. The purpose of this chapter is to address the issue of "craft," or that business of solid preparation for making a living for yourself, and perhaps your children.

In the previous chapter, *Making the Frame*, you constructed a frame for your career and life plan. In fact, you spun a web, a vision of the future for yourself. Without this vision it is almost impossible to face the process of stretching the self. The vision of *The Dinner Party* preceded the stretching of *The Dinner Party* linen over the specially constructed adjustable frames. Chicago (1980, p. 16) describes it as "an extraordinarily tedious and exacting task." But this level of attention to detail and to craft is worthy of the vision, the values expressed in *The Dinner Party*. Is your life any less? Doesn't your career and life plan deserve your attention to detail and to the crafting of a solid foundation so that your vision, your life's purpose is expressed with all the beauty and splendor of the images embroidered on *The Dinner Party* runners? The beauty and splendor of the images could not have been revealed unless *The Dinner Party* linen had been stretched perfectly.

Each runner tells the story of the woman it celebrates. The needlework places the celebrated woman in her historical and cultural context. Similarly, your preparation and your embroidery will reflect your story. The exacting and sometimes tedious work of stretching the self should be understood as an act of celebration, of triumph. You're worth the effort. Your life counts.

The stretching of the self consists of several elements. They are pre-vocational work, vocational testing, research into training and educational opportunities, labor market surveys, money, money, money, and getting the job. Most of the work in this Workbook has been self-reflective, inward, a process of self- knowledge. Now is the time to take this self-awareness into the larger world, to stretch the self.

pre-vocational work

Pre-vocational work is the educational and life preparation usually taken for granted by most people, but is often the educational and life preparation denied to abuse survivors, particularly childhood abuse survivors. Domestic violence, sexual assault, and sex harassment survivors may find that their pre-vocational work is largely about correcting negative worker traits which evolved as a result of post-traumatic stress disorder. Since the average age of entry into prostitution is 13 years, women and girls who are recovering from the prostitution experience may find that they have pre-vocational issues very similar to that of childhood abuse survivors (And, of course, many women and girls used in prostitution have experienced child-hood abuse prior to being used in prostitution.) The exercises you completed in *Understanding Your Vocational Impairment* will provide you with the information you need to decide what pre-vocational work to complete before proceeding to higher levels of education, training, and/or job placement. Some survivors will be able to (or will have to) handle their pre-vocational work simultaneously with going to business college or to graduate school or job hunting.

Return to *Understanding Your Vocational Impairment* in order to complete this exercise.

Three of my most significant negative worker traits are:

1. _____

2. _____

3. _____

I am willing to learn how to manage these negative worker traits.
                    Yes_____ No_____.

negative worker trait pre-vocational work

As we have discovered, post-traumatic stress disorder symptoms and/or negative worker traits can develop as a result of traumatic abuse. There are now many resources for abuse survivors ranging from private psychotherapy to free or low-cost support groups offered by domestic violence shelter agencies (within the shelter and outside of the shelter in community outreach programs) and rape crisis centers. Self-help groups are also available for childhood abuse survivors such as Victims Anonymous. If substance abuse was identified as one of your most significant negative worker traits, 12-Step Programs are available in every city, at all times of the day and night, and can address your substance abuse, the substance abuse of your partner and/or your parents, co-dependency issues, and overeating problems. Books such as Ginny NiCarthy's *Getting Free* for domestic violence survivors, and the Bass and Davis classic *The Courage to Heal* for childhood abuse survivors, are now easily obtained in your local women's bookstore.

What is less available is help in overcoming post-traumatic stress disorder symptoms or complex post-traumatic stress disorder symptoms which are *defined* as vocational impairments or negative worker traits. For example, perhaps you identified an inability to leave the house or inappropriate behaviors in public settings (outbursts of anger, or inability to speak to anyone, or being paralyzed with fear). This is a good example of a negative worker trait because if you can't function in a public setting, how will you ever be able to work in the waged labor force? Happily, many domestic violence shelters, rape crisis centers, women's centers, and women's bookstores unwittingly provide a service which vocational rehabilitation counselors and vocational experts would identify as a form of *work hardening*. Work hardening is a process of being in a safe environment in order to build tolerances and strength. This can be both psychological and physical. A work hardening program is usually set up so that the participant gradually increases her tolerances over a period of time.

Shelter workers nod knowingly at me when I define work hardening for them. They usually tell me a story of a woman who did not need to actually live in the shelter, but needed to come every day to just sit in the office for an hour or two. Inevitably, such women were given work to do just because they were there. In the beginning, these tasks would be very simple (stuffing envelopes for a mailing). Gradually, the woman would relax and begin talking and interacting with the shelter workers and volunteers. Often such women took on more and more responsibility and became recognized volunteers, and sometimes paid staff. The work in a shelter system is both mental and physical, and can involve both exertional and nonexertional activities such as stuffing envelopes and moving donated furniture. Unfortunately, work hardening as a process inside shelter system agencies is a haphazard and unrecognized process and highly dependent upon the personnel who happen to be running the agency at any given time. In my opinion, shelter agencies and rape crisis centers need to be given acknowledgment in the form of funding for the provision of this much-needed service, and I think there should be work hardening specialist paid positions in every domestic violence agency and prostitution recovery center.

Since there is not, it is my recommendation that if you recognize the need for some sort of work hardening process for yourself, design it and do it. The whole world of volunteer work offers itself for such a process. Because you are a volunteer, you can structure how much time you can give, how often you are available, and perhaps, even, what you would like to do. Most communities have lists of volunteering opportunities which can be located in your local newspaper or in the telephone book index under volunteer services. Not only does volunteering lend itself to a work hardening process, it also lends itself to a vocational exploration experience. In other words, it's a way of trying out a vocational goal at no or little risk. Maybe you are interested in landscape design. Volunteering in the community gardens or with the Sierra Club in the building and/or maintenance of trails in parks and forests would give you an excellent idea of the ecological issues embedded in the design of landscapes as well as the physical labor involved. Some volunteering experiences can also be transformed into college course work.

My Work Hardening Process is to: _____

_____

_____

_____

_____

_____

_____

_____

_____

_____

_____

_____

_____

_____

_____

_____

_____

TIP

Remember to put in a timeline (e.g., two hours, twice per week increasing to three hours, twice per week, to 1/2 days on Thursdays and Saturdays).

My lifting limitations are described as follows:

_____

_____

_____

I am willing to either increase my lifting capacity or make certain that my current lifting capacity declines as little as possible as I age, or as my disability progresses.

Yes_____ No_____.

The problems I have with exertional activities are:

_____

_____

_____

I am willing to increase my exertional activity levels or make certain that my current exertional activity levels decline as little as possible as I age, or as my disability progresses.

Yes _____ No_____.

The problems I have with nonexertional activities are:

_____

_____

_____

_____

I am willing to increase my nonexertional activity levels or make certain that my current nonexertional activity levels decline as little as possible as I age, or as my disability progresses. (For survivors with visual and hearing impairments, this may mean learning and/or maintaining mobility skills or sign language proficiency.)

Yes _____ No_____.

Pre-vocational work can also involve improvement of your lifting capacity, and your exertional and nonexertional activity levels. The interaction between your mind and body means that as you overcome or manage your post-traumatic stress disorder and/or negative worker traits, your physical capacity will increase. Conversely, improvement in your overall physical fitness level will give you a better chance of reducing your stress levels. Therefore no matter what your vocational goal may be in the waged or unwaged work worlds, a strong mind and body will allow you to fulfill your goals more easily.

Since the abuse experience is both psychological and physical, it makes sense that recovery should also be both psychological and physical. Work is also physical and psychological, even in those occupations which are defined as sedentary or light work. Therefore neglecting the body in any discussion of vocational planning is not acceptable. Abuse survivors with severe physical injuries, disabilities, and/or pre-existing disabilities will have been confronted with a medical model solution to their injuries and disabilities. This approach may or may not have solved your problems, or have solved your problems somewhat. As we go through health care reform and implementation of the Americans with Disabilities Act, there is an increasing demand that each health care consumer take more and more responsibility for her own health and fitness. The medical model approach does not provide much help since it is based on the notion that an "expert" can "fix" injury and disability, or even worse, that a person with a disability needs to be "fixed." The medical model defines disability and injury in legal systems, insurance reimbursement systems, the Social Security system, and rehabilitation systems. This presents all abuse survivors with a dammed-if-you-do and dammed-if-you-don't problem. You're dammed if you give yourself over to the medical model system to be "fixed," since chances are your inherent worth and dignity, *as you are in your "unfixed state,"* will probably be damaged. But if you don't use the medical model approach, you're dammed because you will not be able to use benefit systems which may be of great importance in your recovery process.

The completion of the exercises in this Workbook will help you maintain your integrity in the face of such contradictions. The development of a written career and life plan placed inside a ten year timeline will allow you use to use these benefit systems without throwing you off the track of *your* life's purpose, not the life purpose someone else (case worker, attorney, rehabilitation counselor) has decided should be your life purpose.

The increasing of and/or maintaining your physical work capacity is also a medical model versus disability rights model issue. That is, you may face such medical model decisions as surgery on your cervical spine to correct an injury caused by battering versus alternative methods of easing pain and increasing flexibility in your neck such as massage or yoga. Perhaps you face taking pain medications and muscle relaxants when you would prefer learning a meditation technique or soaking in a spa daily. Each approach has its merits. I am not suggesting that you should never have surgery or never use pain medications. Nor am I suggesting that yoga, massage, or other body work will "fix" everything. What I am suggesting is that you explore the disability rights approach in managing your disability. That is, you do not hand over your decision-making to the so-called experts. The disability rights approach recognizes that life in a body is a process, not some sort of mechanical event where a unit is removed (perhaps replaced), and the machine is then "fixed." The disability rights approach does not regard the aging body, the body with missing limbs, the body which shakes and trembles, the body whose legs are still, as defective or imperfect. Instead, the notion is that part of everyone's life experience is having a body. Honoring our own bodies at every stage of our lives, in whatever condition our bodies may be in, is an act of reverence, respect, and celebration, not only of ourselves, but for all of life itself.

Abuse survivors know better than most people how to regard our bodies as things or objects because part of our abuse experience(s) has been the use of our bodies by others as things or objects. Therefore, it is my recommendation that survivors explore various bodywork techniques which increase body awareness, and, as a result, a deepening sense of respect and love for our bodies. There are many body awareness techniques which can range from walking daily to taking a Tai Chi class at your local community college or adult education center. If you feel fearful about the more personal bodywork processes such as massage, then start out with activities such as walking or swimming. You may wish to then involve yourself in group exercises such as aerobics, stretch, or yoga classes at your local YWCA or community recreation center. It is very important for all us abuse survivors to experience our bodies in the presence of others. This is because we have learned that being in our bodies in the presence of others is hurtful, shameful. Therefore we need to practice sweating, breathing, flushing, gasping where others can see us and smell us, and *nothing bad happens.*

When you are ready, try massage. I highly recommend massage because it teaches us that even when we are naked and vulnerable we can be safe, that a human hand on our back, our belly, does not mean invasion. We can experience the pleasure of being touched without having to be sexually aroused against our will. If taking off your clothing seems too much, then try your first massages clothed. Trusting the person giving you the massage is very important. If you felt uneasy in the massage because of the person giving you the massage, try somebody else. A massage therapist is as important as a psychotherapist, and just as personal.

Remember that part of the abuse experience is a nonverbal experience. That is, our body takes the abuse in and stores it. Therefore, our recovery cannot be completely verbal, intellectual. It is also physical and emotional. Our feelings have motion. That is, they move between our bodies and our minds. Therefore the pre-vocational work in the stretching of the self will be an exploration of the bodywork we want to do as part of our lifelong recovery process.

For some, the pre-vocational work in increasing your physical work capacity will come out of the medical model. Maybe you've been putting off seeing the doctor, or perhaps you have not been doing those physical therapy exercises to strengthen your back, or maybe you've tossed that medication for your high blood pressure, or maybe you've been drinking and eating mostly candy bars while ignoring that diagnosis of possible diabetes. Maybe you've never had a pap smear or don't give yourself breast examinations. If the medical model intimidates you, then ask for support in confronting it. Have a friend go with you for the pap smear. Insist that she hold your hand when the examination is done.

I have finally faced my own terror of the dentist. I now take my teddy bear, Brownie. Brownie keeps an eye out for sadists who may be lurking in the dentist's office. He rests on my belly during all procedures, and doesn't seem to mind having his stuffing nearly squeezed out of him when the dentist puts the needle into my gums. If I forget to bring Brownie, the staff asks about him. I've met the most charming people in the waiting room when Brownie comes along. Best of all, I no longer have to confess my sad story about how scared I am every time I go to the dentist. Brownie takes care of it all. He is a powerful nonverbal reminder that I require a little extra tender loving care when I go to the dentist.

Feel free to invent your own support systems when confronting the sometimes overwhelming mechanical, drug-infested sphere we now know as going to the doctor, the dentist, the hospital. You have a right to be as comfortable and unafraid as possible.

Putting ourselves in charge when we face the medical model of overcoming limitations and/or impairments to our physical work capacity, and being willing to explore a disability rights approach to managing our limitations and disabilities as a lifelong process through exercise and/or body awareness techniques will automatically improve our physical work capacities.

I will create the following support systems in confronting the medical model approach to increasing my physical work capacity:

_____

_____

_____

_____

_____

_____

_____

_____

_____

_____

_____

_____

_____

TIP

   You may wish to take the information you gathered in *Reclaiming My Innocent Body* and in the "My Physical Work Capacity" from *Understanding My Vocational Impairment* to your doctor, physical therapist, yoga teacher, coach, weight trainer in order to have an informed discussion of how to improve or maintain your lifting, exertional and nonexertional capacities.

_____

I will explore the disability rights approach to improving or maintaining my physical work capacities by:

_____

_____

_____

_____

_____

_____

_____

_____

_____

TIP

A disability rights approach can also include the use of the traditional medical model techniques. The difference is that *you are the expert on your body.*

TIP

A disability rights approach is a life-long approach. That is, the body cannot be "fixed" since it is not a thing. The body is alive and it changes moment by moment. Therefore, we find exercise and body awareness processes which help us stay strong and flexible as our bodies change, age, become vulnerable for whatever reason. Many of us will have lifetime post-traumatic stress disorder. This does not mean that all of our symptoms of trauma will be full-blown all the time. This just means that our trauma symptoms can be triggered. Since trauma is both physical and psychological, it is important to discover physical experiences which strengthen us in our lives just as we discover psychological processes for the same reason (e.g., affirmations, psychotherapy, 12-Step Programs).

TIP

Age and level of disability are not barriers to increasing your physical work capacity. Research has shown that an increase in physical activity for even the most elderly and infirm produces increased mental alertness and well being. The point is, find the activity which is right for you.

This is what I wrote in my journal after I started yoga.

The Woman Pressed Down

The woman was pressed head down, back curved, arms around knees, knees drawn up to the belly, toes curled. She was inside the closet again. Inside the closet, the cubby hole, the space under the staircase, behind the bookcase, under the table, between the bed and wall, by the bush, in a ditch on the side of the road.

She had spent kindergarten in the cloakroom, and the 7th grade in a stall in the Girl's Room. Sometimes, she sleeps this way, on her side, under the covers. She protects her viscera, her innards, her vulva, her breasts.

The trouble is that the neck, the back, and the spine are not happy, and there is a dowager's hump growing between her shoulder blades. When she must uncurl to walk to school, to buy groceries, to work; she does so with heavy hanging head and shoulders tight and high. Now she's having trouble with her feet. Her toes have bunions and corns. She tries to walk without touching the bottoms of her feet to the ground. She has developed a slight lurch, a list in her gait, and this throws her whole body off, and now there is a constant pain under her left shoulder blade. Sometimes, this pain runs down her left arm, and her little finger is numb.

Somehow, the woman gets herself to the yoga master's studio. She cannot remember how she did this, but such laspes are not uncommon for her. She describes it as the holes in the middles of her stories, like the holes in donuts. The yoga master says, "I can cure dowager's hump." The woman's eyelids flash up in disbelief, and down again in hopelessness. The yoga master has small red-blonde braids tightly bound to her skull, and spit curls pasted to her white forehead. The mirrors in the studio reach from floor to ceiling, up a 20 foot wall. The floor is wood, smooth and warm. The yoga master wears a leotard and tights of shiny blue. Her thighs are sculptured muscle, her breasts small, and her movements easy.

"Lift your toes," the yoga master commands. The woman looks down at her crabbed toes. "But I don't know them, not even one of them!" The yoga master is grave. She does not smile. She closes her eyes. Blue eye shadow matches her leotard. "Can you press your toes to the floor, and feel the earth beneath you?"

And so the uncurling began with toes on wood. Smooth warm wood which rose up crying, "Caress me, feel me, stretch, and move yourself all over me!"

And so, the woman did.

As we learned in *Making the Frame*, your educational level has a dramatic effect on your earning potential. Your skill level is tied to your educational level. Therefore, pre-vocational work designed to improve your educational and skill levels is work worth doing.

I identified my educational and skill levels as (see *Understanding My Vocational Impairment)*:

_____

_____

_____

_____

_____

_____

_____

_____

illiteracy

Reading skills seem to be highly vulnerable to traumatic abuse. It is not clear to me why this should be so, and I have not seen any research on this topic. However, I have observed that reading can be associated with childhood abuse by those who were put into closets as punishment for not reading well, or by those who were subjected to other bizarre incidents as children just learning to read. I have also seen adult females convinced that they were not "good" readers by their verbally abusing husbands. In *Making the Connections: Women, Work & Abuse*, a story is recounted in which a husband actually argued with me regarding the testing results which indicated that his wife was, in fact, a superior reader. Perhaps her reading skills meant that she had access to information which was not screened and filtered by this very controlling man.

Reading is a basic skill in our society. It is the foundation of any educational endeavor. Illiteracy is devastating to your chances for increased education and employment. Fortunately, adult literacy programs can be located in most public libraries. It is recommended that you seek out a teacher (often volunteers) whom you like, find easy to talk with, and, ideally, who will be willing to do partner affirmations with you before and after each reading lesson. A suggested affirmation is *I, (name) am safe now*, and/or *My teacher, (name), is here to help me (name)*. Refer back to *Overcoming Verbal-Emotional Abuse* for a refresher on the partner affirmation process.

The need for the affirmation process comes up because the post-traumatic stress disorder symptom of an inability to concentrate or focus may play a key role in the inability to learn to read, to develop good reading skills, or to enjoy reading. Reading requires that we allow the thoughts of the writer to enter our awareness. If we are overwhelmed by obsessive thoughts about our abuse experience, or if we are trying to avoid thinking at all, we may not have the mental space to read. Reading also requires a kind of focus which we may experience as dangerous to us if our survival has been dependent on keeping an eye out for a kick, a slap, or that look on Daddy's face which means only one thing. This is why finding a reading teacher you can trust is so important.

Substance abuse can destroy your ability to read at all, and makes learning to read very difficult, if not impossible. Therefore, if substance abuse, one of the more common side effects of post-traumatic stress disorder, is one of your problems, please understand that attempting to learn to read while abusing substances is probably a waste of your time. Your energy is better spent in 12-Step Programs and verbal support group processes so that you can move toward maintaining the sobriety you need to learn to read.

inability to communicate in english

The inability to communicate in English in American society is an obvious handicap to increasing your skill level, and in obtaining further education. English as a second language programs can be located at low or no cost in most public school systems. The yellow pages in your telephone book list such programs under the category, schools, and sometimes under the subcategory adult education. Although conversational English is essential, literacy in English is also necessary if your goal is to get a high school diploma or go to college.

Immigrant women who have not gained literacy skills in their native languages or in English will be hard pressed to leave violent husbands because the lack of literacy skills in any language generally means a lack of sophistication in dealing with abstract concepts. These women will be at a great disadvantage in making proper decisions for themselves and their children because the dissolution of marriage process is constructed in abstract legal language. Vocational experts providing expert witness testimony and consultation services in such rehabilitative alimony cases should recommend that the divorce settlement be explained to the non-English speaker in her native language. They should also recommend that conversational and literacy skill training in English be provided in any rehabilitative alimony settlement.

marginal education

The obtaining of your high school diploma or passing the General Equivalency Examination (GED) is probably required pre-vocational work for any woman who wishes to get a cosmetology license, enter business college, get a college degree. The high school diploma or GED is a rite of passage into adulthood. Without it, you may feel as though you're driving around without a valid driver's license. The highway patrol or the high school principal patrol will find you out at any moment. It's a kind of looking over your shoulder, an unfinished feeling nagging at you deep inside. All abuse survivors need to experience the completion of things because so much of our lives have been experiences of interruption, delay, and chaos. If your high school diploma was lost in such a shuffle, as a good parent to yourself, you owe it to yourself to finish. And besides, remember the jump in earnings noted in *Making the Frame* — a difference of thousands of dollars per year! Look under schools for adult education telephone numbers in the yellow pages of your telephone book. Make the call today. Classes are usually free. And if you have a criminal record because of being used in prostitution, your high school diploma can be the bridge between your past and your future. It can mean the difference between working and not working.

high school education plus

Many women have hodgepodges of college course work earned as they followed their husbands from job to job, city to city, and even country to country for military wives. If you are one of these women, you may have checked with your state university to see how long it would take you to complete a bachelor's degree. The answer was probably quite discouraging because your course work doesn't transfer, or it doesn't meet the requirements for a traditional degree in business or literature. You were probably told that it would take you three or more years to finish up. It's as though you have done nothing and learned nothing in all those years of travel and in trying to complete your education; as though you are less than the average 18-year-old starting college right out of high school.

Accredited, alternative bachelor degree programs offered by such private institutions as Antioch University and The Union Institute are designed for adults who have some college and who wish to obtain a bachelor's degree. These programs also recognize the wealth of learning adults possess that an 18-year-old could not. Appropriate work and life experiences can be given college credit toward a degree. The senior year of this type of program can be designed to maximize your earning potential upon graduation. In other words, because you have designed your degree for the career goal you have in mind, your degree will not be vague, but meaningful and important to prospective employers. These programs are usually based on student-centered learning. That is, an educational premise which respects the student's learning process. In my experience, students in these programs work much harder than students in traditional degree programs. Since these programs are usually offered by private institutions of higher learning, the tuition costs will appear very expensive when set against the tuition of state supported colleges and universities. However, when you consider the shorter length of time spent in obtaining your degree, because you can transfer most of your earned college credits and work toward credit for work and life experiences, and the longer time you have to earn higher wages as a result of your degree, the costs are probably about the same.

Then there is the second bachelor's degree syndrome which seems to be an affliction of women only. I encountered this syndrome in the late 70s at the Women's

Center at the University of California at Santa Barbara. "Why" I asked myself, "would anybody put themselves through a bachelor's degree twice? Why not just go for a master's degree and do the extra undergraduate course work (if needed) to get into the program?" I have never met a man who decided that he would have to do his bachelor's degree over or get a new one because the degree was decades old, or because he went to college to please his parents, or because he went to college to party, party, party, and play football. Middle class women who went to college to get a man, on the other hand, seem to think that their degree isn't real if their motives weren't pure scholarship. Take it from a vocational expert, the degree is real. Nobody cares about your motives.

If you have never used your degree in the waged labor market, you may have doubts about what you know. If you have been out of the waged labor market for many years and your degree was earned decades ago, chances are you will need some more education. You will probably not need another degree unless you are attempting to enter a professional level occupation which requires advanced degrees such as social worker, counselor, or attorney. If your education was completed prior to the computer technology revolution, you will probably need to become computer literate as soon as possible. Course work is available at your local community college, in extension programs offered by the state college and university systems, and in private business colleges. Certificate programs can be efficient, economical augmentations to a college degree earned years ago. Women who find themselves dumped into the displaced homemaker category may find that such pre-vocational work is absolutely necessary before they can enter the waged job market. A good understanding of how to upgrade an older college degree should be part of your strategy in making any rehabilitative alimony arrangements in a divorce settlement.

My educational level pre-vocational work consists of:

_____

_____

_____

_____

_____

_____

_____

_____

_____

_____

_____

_____

_____

_____

_____

_____

_____

_____

_____

vocational testing

Perhaps you are still not clear about what your skills levels actually are or where your interests are focused. Or perhaps, you are in a system or situation where your aptitudes and interests will have to be documented in order for you to obtain benefits or prove to a judge why you need rehabilitative alimony. For all of these reasons, you may need to be tested. Testing services can be obtained free or at low cost at your local community college career center. These centers will also have self-directed computer search programs which will assist you with completing career exploration exercises.

Most schools require the completion of some sort of entrance examination. These test results can also be used to document your suitability for training and/or your need for training or pre-vocational or remedial work.

Private and public sector rehabilitation counselors, career and life planning experts, and vocational experts also provide testing services. Their expertise is useful in selecting the appropriate tests for each person. For example, a person with limited English or no literacy skills can be tested by using pictorial instruments.

Aptitude testing is designed to help you understand where your skills levels are now. Your reading level, ability to perform mathematical calculations, your perceptual and clerical abilities, your mechanical and spatial skills, spelling and grammar are some of the aptitudes measured. Aptitude test results can be influenced by your mental or physical condition at the time of taking the test. If you have the flu, or have just smoked some crack, had a drink, or find yourself in a panic prior to taking the test, the results will probably not be a true reflection of your aptitudes. It is better to cancel the test than to set yourself up to feel bad about yourself. Aptitude testing should not be regarded as a passing or failing situation, but as a method of vocational exploration. It helps us to answer the question: *What are my aptitudes now? In what areas do I need improvement?* Aptitude testing can help you determine what pre-vocational work you will need to complete before being admitted to a school or training program. It is a valuable tool in your career and life planning kit. If test taking is always a disaster for you, work with your therapist on relaxation techniques. Breathing and the breathing exercise so often referred to in the Workbook can also be helpful prior to and during the testing process.

> **TIP**
> Aptitudes can be changed. That is, for most people, it is possible to improve your reading, your arithmetic, your grammar, your spelling. A suggested affirmation prior to aptitude testing is, I, (name) have the power to improve my aptitudes if I choose to do so.

Curiously, you may be punished for having a high level of aptitudes. This usually occurs when a claims examiner in a workers' compensation system or an ex-husband in a rehabilitative alimony situation doesn't want to pay for an education or training program. You may hear an argument which goes something like this: *Well, she's really smart. So she doesn't need any job training, or further education, because she can just go out and get a job.* **This is simply not true. Never allow**

anyone to confuse you by saying that high scores on aptitude tests mean employability.

For example, you may be a mathematical genius, but if you've never had any computer literacy training or exposure to accounting software programs, chances are no employer is going to hire you. The employer will hire your competitor for the job, the person who has completed the training, has the accounting degree, the certificate in hand. No think tank is going to turn you loose in their mathematical research division without a master's degree or doctoral level training. You may be smartest, but without the training, the credentials, the degrees, you do not have the ticket to ride, to enter the field. A labor market survey which reveals what the minimum requirements are for any given job will provide you with the information you need to justify further education and training. A discussion of the labor market survey process can be located later in this chapter.

And finally, just as we learned in examining our skills in *Analyzing, Respecting and Celebrating Our Work,* that very few people are able to perform every skill at every level, very few people will score at the highest levels on all the aptitude measures. So forgive yourself if your grammar, spelling, and vocabulary are up there in the superior range, but your mathematics scores are somewhere in the basement. It doesn't mean that you are bad or stupid. This just means you need to do some work. Put it on your pre-vocational work list.

Interest testing is, strictly speaking, not testing. It is more of an inventory of your like and dislikes. Interest testing can be very useful in making career choices because, in my professional experience, I have found that skill follows motivation. That is, if you are excited about and interested in something, you are more likely to be willing to go through the hard work and sacrifice it may take to get it. Why bother with the pain of finding out you are not as smart as you thought, or that you need to take remedial mathematics before getting into that accounting class, or that you may have to borrow $10,000 to get your bachelor's degree, if you don't care about your goal? Most of us will simply let it all go, and walk away.

Abuse survivors may experience the post-traumatic stress disorder symptom which produces apathy, a lack of interest in anything, a *why-bother* attitude. Interest testing may help us get around that symptom by giving us clues as to our real interests even though we may not be able to *feel* interested. Sometimes, you may have to act as if you were interested even though your feelings about things have been cut off by your experience(s) of abuse. In other words, interest inventories can give you something to hang on to when your inner voice has been stilled. Acting as if we are interested can sometimes restore our passion for work.

> **TIP**
>
> A suggested affirmation here is, *I, (name) have the right to do my work and enjoy it.* You may also wish to find a woman celebrated in *The Dinner Party* who had work similar to yours (or work you would like to do). Research her life and work in order to provide yourself with a role model of how a celebrated woman managed work and children, or struggled with her female role and her passion for her work.

A passion and excitement about work is something we usually attribute to men, not to women. In fact, many women conceal such passion because it is considered unfeminine, or because such feelings in women are not often understood or supported in our culture. Some of us may feel guilty or selfish if we admit to wanting to spend hours at a time in a studio dyeing yarns and weaving rugs, or writing poems, or discovering new comets through our telescopes. *The Dinner Party* celebrates more than 1,000 women in Western Civilization who managed somehow to leap over their guilt, push away their sensations of selfishness, and who gave themselves to their visions, their passions and left their mark on the history of the achievement of women.

Interest inventories should also be consistent with your aptitudes. That is, if your major interests are in occupations which require college degrees, but your aptitude levels are all in the far below average range, this is an issue you should discuss with your therapist, your support group. Most people's aptitudes are consistent with their interests. That is, most of us are pretty realistic about what we can manage in the world of waged work. If your aptitudes are markedly inconsistent with your interests, you have discovered something very important. Such a result may lead to the most important pre-vocational work you will ever do. Perhaps in therapy, you will finally get to understand why your waged work life is not satisfactory, or why you have trouble hanging on to jobs, or why you are not getting the jobs or promotions you think you deserve.

And finally, some cautionary notes on vocational testing. Some universities and colleges have extensive testing programs for which you can pay hundreds of dollars. If such programs do not include counseling and detailed explanations of test results, don't waste your money. You will have just ended up with a pile of colored paper with strange writing all over it. Testing is just one aspect of vocational exploration and career and life planning. It is one tool in the overall process. Sometimes, testing can be abusive and unethical in the hands of unscrupulous or unskilled professionals who will charge outrageous amounts of money to produce an appearance of objective and scientifically sound reports. This may look impressive in a courtroom or in other legal proceedings. For example, I had a personal injury case in which the plaintiff had a lifetime history of illiteracy based on a learning disorder and hearing loss. The file contained testing which had been completed several times over the course of this man's life. The opposing side subjected this plaintiff to hours and hours of unneeded testing which did not produce any new results. The only purpose served was to allow the expert to make some money. The plaintiff, in the meantime, ended up feeling stupid and exhausted. There was no benefit to him whatsoever. You have the right to refuse testing. If you do so, be certain that you understand the consequences of such a decision. Consultation with your attorney is advised.

RESOURCE – Your local community college counseling and career center is an excellent free or lost cost vocational exploration and testing resource. Many career centers will have user-friendly computer programs which will help you with career exploration and provide you with a print-out of the results.

research into educational and training opportunities

I refer you back to the yellow pages in your telephone book under Schools. You will find not only a listing of public schools, including adult education, but also listing of trade schools, business colleges, real estate schools, truck driving schools, and colleges and universities. Set aside an afternoon and call the schools of interest to you and request their college catalogs. Make appointments to take tours of private schools or meet with an admissions counselor. Make appointments to meet with the financial aid counselor. Ask to be taken to the Women's Center and the Disabled Student's Center at the university or college in your area. Your local library or your local college library will have college catalogs from universities and colleges outside your community, in other cities and states. Ask for extension catalogs from universities and colleges offering bachelor degrees and above. These catalogs are usually separate from the regular course work catalogs, and must be requested from the extension office. This is where certificate programs can be found. Community colleges' catalogs, on the other hand, will contain information on how to obtain associate of arts or sciences degrees and/or certificate programs within one catalog.

If the idea of even setting foot on a campus of any sort gives you the shakes, then ask a friend to come with you. Adult Reentry Programs, Women's Centers, and Disabled Student's Centers can all assist you in the transition into learning as an adult. Some formerly battered women have enlisted the help of the Disabled Student Center to get "Fs" removed from their college transcripts because of the bad grades resulting from being battered while trying to complete classes. (For some women, battering can actually increase when enrolled in school.) This is a way of starting fresh, without a poor grade point average from the past to pull you down, and hold you back.

If you are being stalked, discuss this with the staff of the Women's Center and/or the Disabled Student Center in order to determine if the school can assist you with your safety needs and your needs for confidentiality regarding your class schedule, where you park your car. Stalking may be an Americans with Disabilities Act issue in that you have a right to access to educational opportunities. But because there is no case law on this point at this time, it is not clear whether or not an educational institution is obligated to assist you in this way. However, it never hurts to ask, to raise consciousness.

TIP

Never enroll in or send money to a school you have not visited. Photographs can be of anything. Reality is always more informative than some brochure. Make certain that you enroll in schools which have been accredited by the accrediting agencies appropriate to them. Home study programs have very little credibility, and are most likely a waste of your money. Home study programs should not be confused with independent study programs with accredited institutions such as Antioch University or the Union Institute.

Explore other training opportunities in your community through your state employment service, which usually has information on programs designed for special groups. Some examples include programs for people with criminal records, displaced homemaker programs, the Job Training and Partnership Act (JPTA) Programs. The state department of rehabilitation in your state may also be able to provide you with assistance in creating a vocational rehabilitation plan and money to cover the cost of training and tools. They will also have information about programs developed for special groups. Explore training programs possibly offered through Aid For Dependent Children, or welfare programs in your area. Unfortunately, many of these programs have never been adequately funded so that little child care money is available, or only a very few people can participate. However, you may be one of those people.

Think about on-the-job training possibilities and apprenticeship training programs. Some unions offer apprenticeship programs for women. Apprenticeship programs are a method of learning a skilled trade on the job. Sometimes these programs are offered in cosponsorship with a community college. Other on-the-job training opportunities may have to be created by you. It is much easier to convince an employer to take the time and money to teach you on the job if you are enrolled in a college program which will give you credit for the training. Some community colleges have such programs, and alternative degree programs can also grant credit for such opportunities although they may describe such training as internships, rather than on-the-job training.

labor market surveys

Sometimes, our experience of traumatic abuse can distort our thinking to the point that we may find ourselves focused on an unrealistic vocational goal. A labor market survey is a good method of doing a reality check. When you collect information from schools, colleges, universities, and some of the training programs noted previously, ask for information on job placement as well. This should be the first step in your labor market survey process. If a trade or business school does not have this information, you should avoid the place because they are probably in the business of taking your money, and not in the business of providing you with the education and skill training which will get you a job. Colleges and universities may refer you to their career centers and/or their placement offices for graduates.

The classified ads in your local newspaper, particularly on the biggest advertising days, Wednesdays and Sundays, will give you an idea of what jobs are currently available in your area. Your local library will carry newspapers from other major cities. You may use these newspapers to help you in any relocation decisions.

The yellow pages in the telephone book can also be used to call employers in the fields you may be considering. Many people are willing to give you information about their profession. Ask about the educational requirements, work experience needed, earning potential for the job, and opportunities for full-time and part-time work. Larger companies will refer you to personnel. Small businesses will probably have the owner/manager fulfilling these duties.

Visit the personnel offices for the major employers in your area. These offices frequently have job boards or job listings posted in books. Your state employment office will also have a job board and books listing civil service employment opportunities for city, country, state, and federal jobs.

All of these resources can be used to determine whether or not your vocational goal makes any sense in terms of openings and earnings potential. Making a vocational decision without this information is like trying to drive with a blindfold. Guessing is dangerous in both situations. Clear vision is a must.

RESOURCE – *The Economic Consequences of Child Sexual Abuse in Women,* an unpublished dissertation by Batya Hyman of April, 1993, is available from The National Clearinghouse on Child Abuse & Neglect, PO Box 1182, Washington, DC 20013-1182 for around $25.00. This dissertation is a well-documented piece of quantitative research which reveals that childhood sexual abuse can mean loss of earning capacity as adults in the waged labor markets. *The Effects of Violence on Work and Family,* a research project directed by doctoral candidate, Susan Lloyd, with the Center for Urban Affairs and Policy Research at Northwestern University, 2040 Sheridan Road, Evanston, IL 60208-4100, will be complete in June, 1995. A telephone survey of 1,000 randomly selected adult women in the West Humboldt Park area of Chicago is "expected to add significantly to what is know about women's employment, about the impact of male and street violence on individual women's work and family lives, and about the effects of violence on individual behavior and community well-being.

money, money, money

Okay, so you've done your homework. You've identified a school. Your labor market survey indicates that there are jobs to be had. You understand what prevocational work you will need to complete. You've placed all this on your Manage-

---

TIP
Remember that we don't work just for money. We work for pleasure and dignity too. So if the following exercise does not result in a financial gain, this might be a clue to reexamine your career and life plan goals, but it might also mean that you will complete your goals to improve the quality of your life more than for financial reasons. Both quality of life attainment and financial well-being are valid and important life accomplishments.

ment By Objective Career and Life Plan Statement. You've completed the ten-year plan. Where's the money?

If you haven't met with the financial aid counselor at the school yet, now is the time to make the appointment. You need to understand what loans, grants, scholarships, child care allowances, and work study programs you may be awarded. You need to complete the applications for all these possibilities. You need to understand if any of these financial programs will be of assistance to you.

If you haven't completed the exercises on changing your work life expectancy or your projected annual earnings by your current educational levels in *Making the Frame*, the following exercise will demand that you do it now. It is impossible to make an informed decision about taking on a loan or expense to further your career and life planning process without understanding if the risk of the expense is worth the trouble.

Sample Exercise for a 33-year-old Everywoman

Is the Cost of Overcoming My Negative Worker Traits, Increasing My Physical Work Capacity, and Increasing My Current Educational and Skill Levels Justified by the Change in My Worklife Expectancy and Increased Earning Capacity?

1. Overcoming My Negative Worker Traits   **Costs**

    a) *Take parenting classes for three years for $200 per year*   *$600.00*

    b) *12-Step Group for no cost.*   *-0-*

    c) *Psychotherapy (One on one and group) $3,000 per year for two years*   *$6,000.00*

                      Subtotal <u>$6,600.00</u>

2. Increasing My Physical Work Capacity

    a) *Get regular pap smears – $75 per year for 8 years**   *$600.00*

    b) *Join sports club – $300 per year for 8 years**   *$2,400.00*

    *Number of years before educational goal is completed.

                      Subtotal <u>$3,000.00</u>

3. Increasing my Current Educational and Skill Levels

    a) *Tuition over 8 years of school*   *$6,000.00*

    b) *Books total*   *$2,000.00*

    c) *Child care*   *$4,500.00*

    d) *Tools and supplies*   *$1,000.00*

    e) *Job search attire*   *$500.00*

                      Subtotal <u>$15,000.00</u>

                      Total $24,600.00

My current earning capacity today, 12/27/93, is $15,832.00 annually.

If I do not extend my worklife expectancy (see Figure 2 in *Making the Frame*) by increasing my educational and skill level, I will have a projected (number of years) *28* years of "retirement" to plan for.

With completion of the three goals listed above, my projected earning capacity will be *$25,529.00.* (see Figure 3 in *Making the Frame*) annually by the year *2003* (estimated date of obtaining a job after completion of my educational goals).

This is a good investment since her first year of projected earning capacity after the completion of her goals exceeds her expenses. Her earning capacity has increased by almost $10,000 annually, and her worklife expectancy is extended. (Note: No living expenses were included in this analysis.)

Is the Cost of Overcoming My Negative Worker Traits, Increasing My Physical Work Capacity, and Increasing My Current Educational and Skill Levels Justified by the Change in My Worklife Expectancy and Increased Earning Capacity?

1. Overcoming My Negative Worker Traits: **Costs**

    a) _____   _____

    b) _____   _____

    c) _____   _____

    d) _____   _____

                                              Subtotal _____

2. Increasing My Physical Work Capacity

    a) _____   _____

    b) _____   _____

    c) _____   _____

    d) _____   _____

                                              Subtotal _____

3. Increasing my Current Educational and Skill Levels

    a) Tuition _____   _____

    b) Books _____   _____

    c) Child Care _____   _____

    d) Tools _____   _____

    e) Uniforms _____   _____

f) Job search attire _____   _____

g) Other _____   _____

Subtotal _____

Total _____

My current earning capacity today $ _____ (today's date) is (either list what you earn now or look at the Table 8 (See Figure 3) in *Making the Frame* for an estimate of your earning capacity by your current educational level) $_____ annually.

If I do not extend my worklife expectancy (Table A-5 in *Making the Frame*) by increasing my educational and skill level, I will have a projected (number of years)_____ years of "retirement" to plan for.

With completion of the three goals listed above, my projected earning capacity will be $_____ (see Figure 3 in *Making the Frame*) annually by the year _____ (estimated date of obtaining a job after completion of your educational goals).

This is a good financial investment because:

_____

_____

_____

This is a good quality of life investment because:

_____

_____

_____

_____

_____

The exercise you have just completed does not include money in the form of scholarships, grants, awards from lawsuits, spousal support in the form of rehabilitative alimony, or money from rehabilitation benefit systems. If such money had been available to the woman in the sample exercise, her financial justification for increasing her educational and skill level, and for her other expenses, would have been even better. However, it is most likely that the woman in the sample exercise borrowed money in a student loan program, or from her parents, or through her credit union. You too will most likely face borrowing money in order to accomplish your goals.

The risk of borrowing money often seems overwhelming to most women. In fact, when the Small Business Administration (SBA) set up an outreach program for women in the 70s, they had to redefine what they termed a "small" loan into what is now called a "mini" loan. The SBA defined a small loan as ranging from $100,000 to $1,000,000. They now offer loans as low as $20,000. By the 80s, a whole new concept of start-up loans ranging in the hundreds to thousands of dollars emerged. These are the microenterprise loans which allow women, and other groups outside of the mainstream economic system, to borrow small amounts of money to start or expand small businesses.

If money is a difficult subject for you to handle, or if you find that when you try to think about money, your mind slides away to almost any other topic, or if you find yourself getting very sleepy when the topic of money is raised; then it is probably time to check the community services workshops in your community college course schedule. Enroll in any class that has something to do with money. Such classes or workshops as financial planning, retirement planning, accounting for non-accountants, money management for women, estate planning, management of a stock portfolio, and buying your first home will introduce you to an aspect of the world of money. Taking such classes with a member of your support group, a woman friend, your sister, is a good strategy since you can help each other in avoiding dropping out.

If having a passion for your work is unfeminine, having an interest in money seems to be tantamount to declaring war on the male gender. Some of my most frustrating moments as a counselor have occurred when I've attempted to discuss money with women. Seemingly straightforward questions, *How much money do you need? For child care? Dental care? Health insurance? Housing? Food? Credit card debt?* are greeted with lowered eyes, chair squirming, mumbles. After some such sessions, I've been known to do a little mumbling myself; *Does she think I'm asking her to kill three people on her way to the top?* And, in fact, many women are justifiably fearful of taking on male methods and values in making money, and are afraid of losing their attractiveness to men if they do make more money than they need to support themselves at a minimal level.

In other words, many women don't think they *deserve* to have their own money. Prostitution survivors using the services of the Council for Prostitution Alternatives in Portland, Oregon are given fanny packs upon their entry into the program. This is because women used in prostitution have a difficult time hanging on to their money.

They "lose" it. My theory is that this is a survival technique for women who must hand over their money to their pimps as quickly as possible, and who risk being beaten up for their money by pimps, johns and/or police.

Sex harassment on the job and in education is a method by which women are told that their desires to have money of their own, let alone lots of it and maybe more than some men, are unacceptable and will be punished. Sex harassment is where one of the battlefields between women and men over money, work, and power is located.

The other major battlefield is, of course, marriage and its companion, divorce. The divorce process is largely about two issues. One is the custody of the children, and the other is the division of assets, or who gets what. In today's divorce court, judges assume that women will work in the waged labor market as well as provide child care and housework duties. This means that more than ever before women need to educate themselves about money and the power of having our own money. Our failure to do so not only impoverishes the lives of our children, but of our children's children.

This is because we have not yet learned how the power of money can be used to create institutions which will transmit values important to us. For example, if women cannot raise the money to house *The Dinner Party*, then the generations who follow us will be the poorer because they will have to reinvent the history of women's achievements instead of adding to it. The campaign to build a museum to house this massive artwork has just begun. Leaders have already been cautioned to not frighten women by asking for money too soon, or too loudly. We have been told to not use statements like *$10 million dollars to get started* and *the really big money we need is for the endowment to maintain The Dinner Party Museum.*

But to have money is to have power. The power to buy a house, to get an education, to provide for the education of your children, to control your time, to take vacations, to have a life free from want and fear, to have the power to pass your values on through institutions you create such as *The Dinner Party Museum.* To have money is to do more than "somehow get along," it is to take your rightful place in the world as an adult. A suggested affirmation is, *I, (name) deserve prosperity, and the power, pleasure, and responsibility which comes with it.* If you are taking the risk of borrowing money, a suggested affirmation is, *I, (name) have the right to borrow money because I have the power to repay it.*

getting the job

Employability is based upon a combination of factors including educational and skill levels, positive worker traits, the physical and mental capacity to perform the duties of the job, and current labor market conditions. External factors such as discrimination based on disability, age, gender, race, and sexual orientation may also influence employability. Discrimination is, of course, illegal. It's also tricky. That is, it is sometimes hard to determine if the reason you didn't get the job is because of one of your personal characteristics (worker traits), lack of education or skill level, or because you are in one the groups discriminated against in our society. Abuse survivors who have revealed their histories may find themselves condescended to in a sort of *there-there* sympathy routine which leaves us feels as we've just been patted on the tops of our heads like pound dogs. (I actually had a psychotherapist, who should have known better, pat me on the top of my head. I wanted to bite her.) In other words, discrimination against abuse survivors may take the form of false sympathy and discounting. If you are on the path of developing your full vocational potential (in waged and unwaged work), then your ability to distinguish between discrimination against you because you are a member of a group and you as an individual will be sharper, more focused.

There are days, however, when it feels as though life has been slapping us around. And, in fact, there are things beyond our control such as discrimination and abuse. The eradication of discrimination and abuse does not lay in our personal solutions to our personal experiences. It is only when our personal experiences and personal solutions have meaning and impact beyond our own lives that change can begin. This is why the Workbook material has been designed to continually bring you back to your position within the history of women's achievements and the obstacles yet before us.

What we can do, we must. We do for the sake of ourselves, our children, for other women, for our children's children, and for the children of the world. Our career and life planning efforts take place within a larger political context. Therefore, we don't sacrifice the political responsibility we have to the world outside our lives, nor do we sacrifice our personal lives in the name of some abstract political theory. We go for it all. And women do, when women cannot get jobs, they create them. Women are the small business owners of this nation, and every year we create more new jobs than all the Fortune 500 Companies put together. Necessity is the mother of invention, after all. Who knows this better than we do?

Although the Workbook has not provided much discussion of self-employment, don't overlook this possibility for yourself. Your local community college (that trusty resource) will have workshops, classes, and seminars in starting and operating a small business. Your local Chamber of Commerce will also offer workshops in small business start-up and operation for a minimal fee. They also house the Senior Core of Retired Executive (SCORE) program which consists of volunteers who are willing to consult with you on your dreams for self-employment. I recommend working for someone else in your field of interest while you are developing your small business plan. This is a way to get to paid while learning how to run that business.

Resume preparation and job search skill training are also available through community colleges one-day workshops. Your educational facility may provide these services as part of the training experience, and most colleges and universities have placement offices with counselors who will help you set up interviews, discover job leads, and assist you in preparing a resume. These services are generally free to enrolled students. State employment offices frequently have similar services for job seekers.

In the next chapter, we will explore the use of vocational plans within rehabilitation systems such as workers' compensation, state departments of rehabilitation, welfare systems. We will also discover that some survivors use legal systems as part of their own recovery process, and also to challenge discrimination. Vocational plans play a part in legal systems too.

Whenever we find ourselves inside of the modern bureaucratic state and its various systems, we are confronted with the excruciating process of trying to connect and disconnect our personal lives to and from these systems. Unfortunately, these systems were not created by women to meet their needs. They were created by men to meet their needs. This means, as women, we are always in a process of inventing ourselves, of designing our lives. The last chapter is titled, *Weaving A Life*, because unless we have become skillful weavers, we will be run over by the modern bureaucratic state which is patriarchal to the core. That is, as you have completed the work in this Workbook, you have learned how to make a life for yourself, and you will be able to weave and reweave the patriarchal systems into your pattern, for your own benefit, and by so doing, challenge and change them.

Congratulations!

thirteen

----

weaving a life

The technical problems to be solved in order to properly interpret
Chicago's cartoon were sobering. The cartoon was incredibly de-
tailed, and Chicago wanted the beauty and delicacy of those details
translated into tapestry. I had never worked in such fine detail be-
fore and found the slowness of the work frightening at first. I was
concerned that I might not be able to complete the piece on time. As
the weaving progressed, however, and I saw that it was just as gor-
geous as Chicago and I had hoped, my excitement grew.

Audrey Cowan from Judy Chicago, 1980, p. 142

Perhaps one of the most devastating results of the pandemic levels of traumatic
abuse experienced by the world's women and girls has been our isolation from each
other and our achievements. This has meant that we are always reinventing the wheel
instead of "standing on the shoulders of giants," as the history of the achievement of
men is often described. That is, men keep careful account of their achievements, and
acknowledge the genius on which the next generation can build. So even though
men are competitive with each other in work and accomplishment, they also value
the knowledge of the past and the importance of work with other men in order to
develop themselves fully.

We are not alone, even though as traumatic abuse survivors we may have been
convinced of our unique, defective, and solitary condition. When we move toward
the achievement of excellence in the weaving of our life patterns, we may act to
protect our isolation. If we have managed to obtain an education and some power in
a job setting, we may take on a Queen Bee attitude toward other women who would
like to follow in our footsteps. We may even attempt to derail or destroy the careers
of such women in the name of our own need to be special or unique. Some of us may
maintain our solitary ways to sustain our feelings of false superiority by never join-
ing our professional associations or by scoffing at the women's movement. And
many of us will attack and discredit women we feel are superior to ourselves in
some way. All of these behaviors are self-protective, a way of denying how fright-

ened and alone we feel, how threatened we are that if we do join with other women that we will be found out to be maimed, deformed, not women, maybe not even human.

We may have gone to the other extreme, which is to place ourselves and our trust blindly, expecting a female mentor to be all things to us at all times. The mother we never had. The father who should have taught us how to survive in the world of men. The perfect woman — all forgiving, all embracing, all nurturing, and always available to us. This expectation is, of course, doomed. We can then retreat into our solitary conditions justified in our belief that bonding with other women, and learning from other women is a waste of time. We say, *I don't need anyone.*

The relationships between Judy Chicago and the women who have worked with her over the years in her many collaborative art projects offer a rich resource for us to examine our own isolation, and perhaps our resistance to entering the community of women to whom we belong. Fortunately, these relationships are explored in all of Chicago's books as a subtext, running like a vein of gold throughout.

Audrey Cowan's comments, about weaving a cartoon created by Chicago, are instructive for all of us who have experienced the shattering of our trust, the underlying tragedy of all traumatic abuse. Cowan describes herself as frightened and sobered by the task before her. She writes that she "had never worked in such fine detail before." The slowness of her work process alarms her. She doesn't think she will finish in time. In other words, she is assailed by doubt and fear. But she persists. Why? Because she has decided to take a chance, to risk, to trust the vision shared with Chicago. And as "the weaving progressed," her trust was rewarded. "It was just as gorgeous as Chicago and I hoped."

You have taken a similar risk in completing any or all of the exercises in this Workbook. It is not just my vision you are weaving, but a vision which you have created based on your life, the lives of the many women referred to in the Workbook, and the lives you may have discovered in your research. Without this vision before you, as expressed in *Spider Woman's Dream – My Ideal Life* and the synthesis of that – *My Management by Objective Career & Life Plan Statement*, it will be almost impossible for you to trust, to risk in the face of the modern bureaucratic state, the coming up against law, medicine, welfare, rehabilitation, education, and economics. You will be required to manage doubt and fear. You will be dismayed by how long everything takes. You will tell yourself that you've never done technical work before and how could you be expected to understand? But as your weaving progresses, and as you weave and re-weave the challenges your life gives you, it is my dream that your life is as gorgeous as you and I had hoped.

the *take-the-money-and-run principle* of career and life planning weaving

The *Take-the-money-and-run Principle* is based on the sad, but true, fact that most rehabilitative and legal systems are based on blame, control, and even coercion. If you approach any of these systems with the post-traumatic stress disorder symptoms of paranoia and suspicion, or their opposites, blind trust and romantic dependency, you will not be able to use these systems to your advantage. If you think or wish that the workers' compensation system, the welfare systems, the state department of rehabilitation, the new rehabilitative alimony process in divorce, a sexual harassment administrative procedure is going to bring you justice and make up for what has been done to you, you will feel betrayed, and angry, and enraged, and defeated. If you didn't expect anything anyway, and you just knew that all those case workers and rehabilitation counselors were out to do you dirt, then all of your worst expectations will be confirmed.

You need to position yourself firmly in the center of the web you have woven, just as the Goddess has taught us. Center yourself like a golden spider I once saw in a dew-covered web stretched across a forest trail in the High Sierra above Lake Tahoe. The web sparkled in the morning sun and mist, and she glittered there in all her beauty, throwing her threads out to see what she could catch. Center yourself inside your career and life plan within the ten-year timeline. If you do this, you will be able to examine the use of legal and rehabilitative systems will a cold, clear eye. Like the spider, you may ask yourself, *Is this food? Is this good for me? Will I be nurtured? Is this worth the expenditure of my life energy? Can my babies eat this?*

If these questions can be answered to *your* satisfaction, then you will be able to use *Take-the-money-and-run principle of Career & Life Planning Weaving* because you will see legal and rehabilitative systems as food and energy, rather than as systems to save us, or systems to enslave us.

The only way I survived more than a decade as a rehabilitation counselor in workers' compensation systems was to adopt a process I termed, *sorting out the truth and the facts.* When I did this, my work was easier, and I felt better about myself. My dignity was preserved. This technique should work for you as well.

First, it is important to understand that *all bureaucratic systems* — legal, medical, rehabilitative, welfare, academic — *are based on rules and laws.* These rules and laws are written down in law books, policies and procedure manuals, brochures and pamphlets. All of this material is then interpreted by human beings, most of whom were not there when the stuff was written down, and who have no idea what it means. The stuff written down was usually fought over in a legislative session, or in the governor's office, or in the media (as in the Anita Hill/Clarence Thomas sexual harassment television drama). This means the rules and laws are some sort of compromise which reflect the current political and social attitudes in ascendancy.

The second point is: *They change.* The laws and rules, and how they are interpreted, change. So just when you think you've got it figured out, it's changed. This means you might get your checks on the 5th and 20th of the month, instead of the 1st and the 15th, which plays hell with your ability to keep your landlord happy and the kids' bellies full. In my 16-year career in workers' compensation systems, I have been through three major reforms of the workers' compensation vocational rehabilitation benefit system in two states. *Changes affect everybody in a system, and not just the person to whom the benefit is to be delivered.* In other words, if you think you're confused, you are not alone. So is everybody else.

The third thing to remember is: *It's not personal.* It's certainly *feels* that way as in, *"What do you mean my claims examiner went on vacation, and that's why my check was never mailed?"* You have every right to be outraged at such treatment, but such a failure in the system is truly not personal. Most systems have no interest in you as an individual at all. Bureaucratic systems mindlessly grind on like some sort of perpetual motion machine. Your personal needs, feelings, and desires have nothing to do with the needs and desires of the system. Bureaucratic systems do not have feelings. It is not the nature of the beast.

And now we come to *sorting out the truth and the facts. Bureaucratic systems operate on facts only.* Their operation has nothing to do with the truth, absolutely nothing. What I mean by this is that *facts* are the sets of rules or laws currently being used to drive a particular system. If you use these rules and laws and the language or current buzzwords to operate within the system, you will make progress. (Remember that progress means taking the money and running.) If you try to get messy with the truth, the system will break down or punish you. Either way, you won't get the money.

I am not suggesting that you neglect the *truth*. The *truth* in any bureaucratic system is the human interaction you have in that system with *anyone* in the system. The difference between human beings and bureaucratic systems is that human have feelings, needs, and desires. Systems don't have feelings. They are driven by needs and desires. (Usually, the need to survive and the desire to be bigger than they are now.) The *truth* is also what you tell yourself about what you want from the system.

Sorting the truth and the facts means that when you are dealing with a human being, either by telephone or in person, you make every effort to be present. That is, you are aware of this human being as an individual. You are aware of the tone of voice, the color of her hair, what she is wearing today. Is she happy? Sad? Is there something different about her today? You communicate your humanness to her, and you allow her to see yours. You make the case worker, the attorney, your buddy inside the system. You will notice I used the word *buddy* rather than the word *friend*. These folks are not your friends, because they are inside a role or a position used by the system to get things done. They cannot be your friend, but they can be your buddy, your advocate inside the system. And you can be a buddy to them in the sense of we-are-all-in-this-together, which is true, and is *truth*.

The facts then become the language of the rule and the laws of the system. The job of the counselor or caseworker or attorney is to implement or enforce these rules and laws. So play the game with them. Become the golden spider with her cold eyes. Stay in the center of your web. *How do I do it? What information do you need? Can you show me some examples of how others have done it?*

> **TIP**
> Remember that bureaucratic systems rest upon *written* information. Therefore, anything in writing should be formulated as facts using the language of that system. This is because bureaucratic systems document everything so that they can justify their existence. Truth has no need for justification, and so is more fleeting, ephemeral. Within bureaucratic systems, truth usually shows up in conversation.

Do you recommend any particular way of filling out this form? Are there any road-blocks I should look out for? Do you recommend that I discuss my career and life plan with the counselor rather than giving *it to her in written form?*

One truth women avoid is admitting that they want, need, and maybe even, enjoy having money. The sex-role stereotyping around money is so potent that women still have a hard time talking about money in relationship to themselves. The association between a woman's sexuality and money is always the woman as whore, and the move toward the further legalization of prostitution is always justified by the idea that women can make lots of money by being used in prostitution. Prostitution survivors, on the other hand, laugh at the moralistic swooning lady who can't handle the idea of herself and money in the same thought.

The problem with all this is that our denial of our needs, wants, and pleasures in having our own money leads us into all sorts of lies and blather. If you find yourself in a benefit system saying something like, *"It's not the money. It's the principle, you know?"* Please. Spare me. Spare yourself. Spare your caseworker, your counselor. Of course, it's the money! It had damn well better be the money. Don't you have to eat? Pay the rent? Buy clothes for the kids?

Take a deep breath. Only Queen Elizabeth gets to go around without money in her purse. We are not ladies. The prince is not going to show up. And we are not available to be used in prostitution of any sort to justify our need, desire, and pleasure in money either.

> **TIP**
> A suggested affirmation is, *I, (name) deserve to have my own money.*

And sometimes, nothing works. That is, some caseworkers, attorneys, rehabilitation counselors, claims examiners have become the system. They've lost their feelings, and they are left with needs and desires. Sometimes, it is possible to ask for and get another caseworker or attorney or counselor. Sometimes, like the cold-eyed spider you will examine what's in your web and decide, *I can't eat that.* She snips the threads and the offending, unnourishing thing drops away. Sometimes, it's better to cut our losses, and walk away.

And sometimes, especially with a lawsuit, we proceed not for money, but for justice, for the opportunity to make a statement, as part of our healing process. Such decisions should be weighed very carefully in terms of their consequences.

What I want out of this benefit system (lawsuit, procedure) is:

_____

_____

_____

_____

_____

_____

_____

The way I can use this benefit system (lawsuit, procedure) in my Career & Life Plan Weaving is:

_____

_____

_____

_____

_____

_____

_____

_____

Once you understand what it is you want from a system, and how it fits into your career and life plan weaving, you will be in a much better position to take the money and run. Or, sometimes, just run.

What follows are some guidelines in handling particular legal and rehabilitative systems. Not every system can be addressed within the scope of this Workbook, but perhaps some of the tools you have learned to use here will help you in all of them.

Women are still in the process of inventing themselves, defining themselves from their own point of view. Some feminists refer to the Women's Movement of the 60s and 70s as the Second Wave, and the increasingly complex discussions of what the word *woman* means as the Third Wave. The Third Wave probably started somewhere in the 80s and is still with us. The First Wave refers to the suffragists' efforts in England and the United States in the early part of this century.

Part of the Third Wave discussions center on an emerging field of study known as *feminist jurisprudence*. This is a multifaceted body of knowledge which has exploded since the late 70s. We now have not only criminal legal proceedings such as temporary restraining orders against stalkers and batterers and rape reform laws which have resulted in increased conviction rates against rapists, but also an emerging body of civil law including domestic torts, civil sexual assault, civil incest, sex discrimination and sexual harassment law. New laws are being proposed. The Violence Against Women Act will, for the first time, allow women to bring civil lawsuits against those who have committed violence against them based on their gender. This is the first hate crimes bill based on gender.

Perhaps the whole body of employment law reveals the influence of the Third Wave of the Women's Movement more than any other, because employment discrimination law is based not only on gender, but also race, ethnicity, and age. The Third Wave focuses on diversity as a correction to the often racist reduction of the word *woman* to mean *white woman* as the paradigm for what a woman was, is, should be. The newly formed National Employment Lawyer's Association's proceedings from their 1992 convention reads like advanced graduate courses in women's studies, ethnic studies, and disability studies. The interdisciplinary character of the legal theories communicated in this enormous document is astounding in its range, variety, and number of disciplines. All of these emerging bodies of law and judicial theory then act to change more traditional, patriarchally-based law such as workers' compensation law, and the laws which regulate various benefit systems such as Social Security Disability Insurance, federal rehabilitation benefit law, and veteran's benefits. It will be exciting to see how the 1990 Americans with Disabilities Act implementation is influenced by feminist jurisprudence concepts.

Perhaps no body of law has been more influenced by the emergence of women in our society than divorce law, and since divorce law is probably what most of us will encounter sometime in our lives, we will start there.

the rehabilitative alimony support plan in the dissolution of marriage and domestic tort processes

No-fault divorce started in California and swept the nation in divorce law reform in the 60s and 70s. Since that time, there has been a presumption by the courts that women who are able to work in the waged labor market will do so. In 1980, California allowed either the supported spouse or the spouse providing spousal support to use the services of vocational experts to provide vocational evaluations, and to present rehabilitative alimony support plans. Other states have followed (e.g., Nevada in 1989 and New Mexico in 1993).

For the first time, vocational rehabilitation professionals were forced to examine the work lives of women in light of a family law perspective. This perspective made it more difficult to evaluate women as some sort of deviant men, as is usually done in traditional rehabilitation systems. This does not mean that most vocational experts will now provide vocational evaluations from a women-centered point of view. In fact, vocational rehabilitation graduate training programs have scarcely been touched by women's studies and feminist jurisprudence. Therefore without a career and life plan of your own, you may end up with a vocational evaluation which ignores or discounts the time it takes to provide quality child care. You may find yourself expected to work for minimum wages and be the primary caretaking parent with no foreseeable increase in your earning capacity or standard of living for the future. Your needs for retirement planning may be completely overlooked.

Many private sector rehabilitation counselors are accustomed to working with claims examiners and industrially injured workers. This creates a mind-set where, in a divorce case, the counselor may view you, the supported spouse, as the injured worker and your ex-husband as the insurance carrier or the employer. This can lead to a vocational plan where money for education is awarded to you on a class by class basis in the name of some sort of accountability. I have had cases where the ex-husband also wanted to be able to determine what classes his ex-wife would take! You are not an injured worker, and your husband is not your employer, and a dissolution of marriage process is not workers' compensation. You have the right to your vocational aspirations. You have the right to determine how, where, and when you will fulfill these aspirations.

> **TIP**
> The Workbook can be used by you as a check on the vocational expert either hired by yourself, your husband, or appointed by the Court. Responsible and ethical experts will welcome your active participation in the process of determining what you will require in rehabilitative alimony support. The best method is to try for a win-win situation. The establishment of your highest earning potential is not only good for you (and your children), but also for your ex-husband since he will not have the burden of providing alimony after your vocational endeavors are completed.

If you are a domestic violence survivor leaving a longtime marriage, you may find yourself completely confused and overwhelmed by the sudden demand that you go to work in the waged labor market. This may be because you married young and were told that your primary role was that of wife and mother. You may have been punished for working or for going to school. You may have even had your life threatened when you expressed a desire to work.

If you did work for wages, you may have been driven to work by your husband, and picked up at the end of the day. You may have had to account for your activities during the workday by reporting to your husband throughout the day by telephone and/or after your work day was over. You may have had to account for how your time was spent, with whom, and why. You may have lost jobs because of your husband's behaviors. You may have come into work with visible bruises, and been fired as a result, or endured the humiliation of your experience in front of your supervisor and your co-workers. You may have worked at the same company as your husband. This then allowed him to keep track of you in person. You may have been stalked by a husband, boyfriend, or ex-husband in the workplace by his getting a transfer to your new location or department, or by his waiting for you in the parking lot, or calling you on the telephone continually. All of these experiences damage your vocational potential, and should not be ignored in any vocational evaluation leading to a rehabilitative alimony award.

Women who have had histories of domestic violence lasting as long as the marriage, and who have had little or no waged work history, and who married very young may find that their vocational maturity or work identity development may be where it was at the time of the marriage. In other words, they may find themselves with the work identity development of an 18- or 20-year-old even though they are now 43 or 52 years of age. This may mean the need for several months to a year or more of vocational exploration, and perhaps work hardening, before an informed decision can be made about vocational directions or goals. After all, isn't this the process young adults undergo upon their graduation from high school? They take general education classes, or travel, or try out jobs before settling into a major or into more permanent work. They are given time to explore so that they can make informed decisions about their futures.

If this is your situation, you may find that judges, attorneys (even yours), and your ex-husband may find your need for such vocational exploration time to be unusual, even outrageous. In my experience, women who needed this vocational exploration time usually ended up taking it whether or not it was recognized in the rehabilitative alimony award. Such women lost their rehabilitative alimony, or portions of it, as a result. The cost of a vocational expert may be well worth the expense in these situations. A vocational expert who is well-grounded in women's work patterns and the vocational impairment caused by domestic violence can be of great assistance to you in such a situation. The expert can explain career maturity and work identity development to judges, attorneys, and your ex-husband.

This period of vocational exploration will need to be accompanied by traumatic abuse recovery efforts which can mean psychotherapy, support group attendance, and 12-Step Programs. These costs should also be included in the rehabilitative alimony support award. Women with a defined goal may also need their recovery expenses covered as part of a complete vocational rehabilitation process.

> **TIP**
>
> Women who are identified by the Courts as battered women have lost custody of their children because they are battered women! Women who don't appear to have much in the way of earning capacity have also lost custody because the father has more money. In both situations, your comprehensive career and life plan will be your best defense, and may be very important in your ability to keep your children with you. A suggested affirmation is, *I, (name) have the power to create a new life for myself and my children.*

> **TIP**
>
> If you are a woman whose husband will not or cannot provide rehabilitative alimony, don't think that the work of creating your career and life plan is useless. A comprehensive career and life plan will still be useful to you in custody issues and in work programs located in welfare systems, if AFDC is what you are facing. Your plan will also be a valuable tool for the domestic violence agency you may be working with to assist you in getting grants, on-the-job training, transitional housing, and other benefits. In other words, the power of presenting yourself as the responsible, dignified adult that you are should not be underestimated. A suggested affirmation is, *I, (name) have the power to create a new life for myself and my children.*

Once divorce became a no-fault process, battered women were left without any recourse in the divorce courts. As a result, a new body of law called *domestic torts* has evolved. These laws allow husbands and wives to sue each other in civil court for damage awards. The domestic tort is a very important tool for battered wives whose traumatic abuse has resulted in psychological and/or physical disability. Each state in the United States is evolving laws regarding domestic torts either through case law (law which comes through the courts) or by legislation. Each state has its own laws about the relationships between the dissolution of marriage process and the domestic tort process. In some states, you will be required to indicate your intention to file a domestic tort in your divorce settlement.

Some states do not allow testimony regarding domestic violence issues and rehabilitative alimony support plans, and others do. In some states you may not wish to, or need to, file a domestic tort since your needs can be handled in the divorce court. In other states, your only recourse is to file a domestic tort along with the dissolution of marriage process.

Domestic torts are still very difficult to bring forward because most attorneys are not yet knowledgeable about this new body of law, because there are few experts available to assist attorneys in developing these cases, and because the injury and vocational impairment which results from battering are still not understood in our society. A woman who has the courage to go forward with a domestic tort is a hero. Her actions break new ground for the attorneys who represent and oppose her, for the experts who attempt to explain her, and for the women who follow her. Some women use the legal system as part of their recovery process. They are daring weavers.

TIP

It is not my intention to urge you to file a domestic tort. This decision can only be reached by each person after careful thought and consultation with the appropriate experts – attorneys, vocational experts, therapists. However, your decision to **not** file a domestic tort should also be carefully considered.

A comprehensive vocational plan which identifies the vocational impairment caused by battering can be a powerful tool in dissolution of marriage settlement negotiations. And just the threat of a domestic tort can sometimes bring about a just and fair spousal support or rehabilitative alimony award. Be certain that you clearly understand your options, because you may have only one chance to make a decision regarding a domestic tort lawsuit.

It is assumed that you have completed the work in this Workbook, that you have developed a career and life plan set inside a ten-year timeline, and that you have consulted with your attorney regarding the legal issues in your dissolution of marriage and/or domestic tort case prior to using the sample below and filling out the worksheet for your own use.

The following Sample Rehabilitative Alimony Support Plan is exactly that, a sample. It, and the blank worksheet which accompanies it on the next pages, are meant to be suggestions only. This is because I have no way to design a form for each situation in all of the 50 states. Your attorney will be able to advise you and your vocational expert how such plans need to be tailored according to the laws in your state. The work you have completed in this Workbook will allow you to extract the information you need to create a form or worksheet of your own.

Sample Three and 1/2 Year Rehabilitative Alimony Support Plan in the Dissolution of Marriage (& Domestic Tort Processes)

INJURY/DISABILITY	RECOVERY PROCESS	TIMELINE*	MONTHLY COST	TOTAL COST
Post-traumatic Stress Disorder	psychotherapy support group	years 1 and 2 years 1, 2, and 3	$300.00 -0-	$7200.00 -0-
Neck injury	chiropractic yoga classes	1st year 1st year	$200.00 $100.00	$2400.00 $1200.00
Loss of right eye	Surgery, new glasses	completed	to be arranged	$5565.00

VOCATIONAL IMPAIRMENT	PRE-VOCATIONAL WORK	TIMELINE*	MONTHLY COST	TOTAL COST

The First Year

VOCATIONAL IMPAIRMENT	PRE-VOCATIONAL WORK	TIMELINE*	MONTHLY COST	TOTAL COST
Fearful and shy in public	Work hardening through volunteering	6 months	-0-	-0-
Confused about vocational goals.	Work with vocational expert or career and life counselor	6 months	$250.00	$1500.00
No significant waged work history.	Vocational exploration by taking classes, workshops.	within 1st year	allowance of $500.00 to draw upon	
Child care expenses while in work hardening, vocational exploration, and traumatic abuse recovery.		1/2 days for 12 months	$300.00	$3,600.00

The Second and Third Years

VOCATIONAL IMPAIRMENT	TRAINING	TIMELINE*	TUITION PER TERM COST	TOTAL COST
No skills, training, degrees, or certificates to sell in waged labor market.	Start AA degree in business.	2 years start on Fall, 19 __ and complete Spring, 19__.	$300 for 4 terms (includes books and supplies).	$1,200.00
Child care expenses while in school and for study time at school.		2 years as above and during job search of 6 months.	At college, day care center costs are $150 monthly for 1/2 days.	$4,500.00

Spousal Support and Child Support

Spousal Support from present to six months after graduation from college with A.A. degree. $1,500 monthly for 42 months is $63,000.00.

Child Support as agreed with child care expenses above and beyond child support during the 42 months of the Rehabilitative Alimony Support Plan.

*Timelines are variable. You will need to insert dates, or set up timelines according to the logic of your plan (e.g., your school is on the quarter system).

My _____ Year Rehabilitative Alimony Support Plan in the Dissolution of Marriage (& Domestic Tort Processes)

INJURY/DISABILITY	RECOVERY PROCESS	TIMELINE*	MONTHLY COST	TOTAL COST

The First Year

VOCATIONAL IMPAIRMENT	PRE-VOCATIONAL WORK	TIMELINE*	MONTHLY COST	TOTAL COST

The Second Year

VOCATIONAL IMPAIRMENT	TRAINING	TIMELINE*	TUITION PER TERM COST	TOTAL COST

The Third Year

VOCATIONAL IMPAIRMENT	TRAINING	TIMELINE*	TUITION PER TERM COST	TOTAL COST

The Fourth Year

VOCATIONAL IMPAIRMENT	TRAINING	TIMELINE*	TUITION PER TERM COST	TOTAL COST

The Fifth Year

VOCATIONAL IMPAIRMENT	TRAINING	TIMELINE*	TUITION PER TERM COST	TOTAL COST

Spousal Support and Child Support

The rehabilitative alimony plan should be accompanied by a narrative report which would summarize the overall monthly and total costs to the supporting spouse. In some dissolution of marriage settlements, a lump sum award is given to cover these costs (perhaps by selling a house or some other property). In that case, you will have succeeded in creating budget for yourself to follow in the use of your lump sum settlement.

Supporting documentation such as a labor market survey which backs up the availability of jobs and the wages paid, and college catalogs and course schedules should be available if the court wants that information, or if you think your estimates are going to be challenged by your ex-husband's attorney.

Medical and psychological reports documenting physical and physical injuries will be essential supporting documents for your rehabilitative alimony plan. You may also have to bring in fee schedules for child care expenses and/or a written letter from your baby-sitter regarding her fees.

> **TIP**
>
> Awards for emotional distress damages can also be granted in domestic torts if the state laws allow it. Such awards are not given in no-fault divorce settlements. The rehabilitative alimony plan worksheets do not include such damages. A discussion of noneconomic awards such as emotional distress will be discussed later in this chapter.

> **TIP**
>
> Most judges and court systems are overwhelmed. Therefore the easier you can make it for the judge to understand what it is you need, what your justification is for needing it, and how much it will cost, the more likely you are to get exactly what you want. In one divorce case, a judge picked up the term "machine" to refer to a computer system (computer, printer, monitor, keyboard, software, cables). The ex-husband used the word "machine" to justify buying a computer only. The ex-wife was forced to return to court to get an entire system, which she needed to start her own graphic design free lance practice.

You will have noticed that the worksheet above does not cover your Management by Objective Career and Life Plan Statement set inside your Ten-year timeline. This will be true for whatever worksheets you will use in legal and rehabilitative systems. It is unrealistic to think that any one person (your ex-husband), or any one system or institution (welfare, workers' compensation, college loans and grants) will take you through your entire Ten-year timeline. The reason for having a ten-year span of time to think about is to prevent you from returning to the trap of that old marriage plot. Remember the song? *Somehow I'll just get along, and someday my prince will come.* Our old conditioning to be dependent will be triggered by finding ourselves inside a bureaucratic system of some sort. If this happens, we will find ourselves resentful, angry, and fearful of the betrayal which is bound to show up sooner or later. If, on the other hand, we sustain our vision of the life we want to weave for ourselves slowly, carefully, with great attention to detail, then we can use these systems without expecting to be rescued or saved by them.

One way to help largely male judges, attorneys, and perhaps, your husband to understand what it takes to raise children and work, or raise children and go to school, or raise children, go to school, and work; is to provide them with an accounting of your typical day hour by hour. It has been my experience that since most men have not had the primary

TIP

Remember the *Take-the-money-and-run principle.* In other words, don't get too comfortable with your alimony, your workers' compensation check, your welfare income. Take what is rightly yours, but always have your plan in mind for independence. And get out as soon as possible!

care of children, they are free to regard child rearing as some sort of strange hobby you insist upon doing. This notion is further supported when the man in question has a hefty earning capacity. These men are able to simply buy child care, and they have a difficult time really understanding what you are saying when you talk about *quality of child care*. There is almost no understanding of the 24-hour-per-day on-call *responsibility* of being the caretaking parent, whether or not you actually had to do something for the child that day. The daily activity log can help all the men in your divorce process understand your concerns. The term *on-call* is very powerful in this context since it was probably invented by male doctors to reflect their responsibility to their patients. It implies that they are not free to be out of touch, and neither are you as the caretaking parent. The daily activity log should accompany your vocational plan.

Sample Daily Activity Log for the 24-hour-per-day On-call Parent

Hour	Activity
6 AM	Get up. Feed the baby. Make breakfast for myself and the boys. Dress baby. Supervise boys getting ready for school. Do breakfast dishes. Make lunches. Prepare dish for dinner.
7 AM	Walk boys to bus stop. Drive baby to baby sitter. Drive to first class at community college.
8 AM	Computer literacy class.
9 AM	Computer Lab
10 AM	Business Communications
11 AM	Stop at dry cleaner's, pick up groceries, put in job application at the state employment office. Drive to baby sitter and pick up baby.
NOON	Change baby. Make telephone calls to pediatrician for inoculations and baby's possible ear infection. Try to get baby to sleep after giving her baby aspirin. Have lunch. Throw a load of wash into the machine. Vacuum the living room.
1 PM	Study for midterm examinations.
2 PM	Change baby. Make telephone calls regarding a new baby sitter. Call school to see if there are any openings or where I am on the waiting list for day care at my school.
3 PM	Get snacks ready for the boys to come home after school. Supervise boy's home work. Put hot dish into the oven. Fold laundry. Try to figure out what to prepare for meals for a few days ahead. Make up these dishes and put in freezer.
4 PM	Study for midterm examinations. Arrange to drop car off at repair shop on Tuesday. Fill out applications for state college, loans, child care, and request transcripts. Call on job leads from the want ads.
5 PM	Feed the kids. Play with the baby. Bathe baby. Supervise the boys in the tub. Get dressed for work. Iron uniforms.
6 PM	Greet baby sitter. Tell her about the baby and baby aspirin. Kiss boys goodnight. Drive to The Dew Drop Inn for the cocktail waitress job.
7 PM	Work the cocktail lounge and answer telephone calls from new baby sitter.
8 PM	Same
9 PM	Same
10 PM	Same
11 PM	Same
MIDNIGHT	Drive home. Pay baby-sitter. Take a bath. Check on baby and boys.
1 AM	Go to bed.

This is my schedule Tuesday through Saturday. On Mondays, I attend school but I don't work. Sunday is my day of rest, but I usually study and attend events to watch my boys in Little League and other sports. The alternative weekends, when the baby and the boys are with their Father, I use for major housework and to catch up on my studies and sleep.

Sample Daily Activity Log for the 24-hour-per-day On-call Parent

Hour	Activity

The daily activity log is often a valuable exercise for you, too. If you have not had to face school and child care, or work and child care issues, or work, school, and child care issues; you will need such a log in order to figure out if you can accomplish all that you wish. This saves biting off more than you can chew, or the alternative may be true. You may be able to do more than you had guessed.

the employment law and workers' compensation law fandango

The relationship between the bodies of law known as employment law and workers' compensation law is a dance dreamed up in some sort of special bureaucratic hell. Sexual harassment survivors may find themselves in *both* systems! And at the same time! One is bad enough.

Workers' compensation law is supposed to be an *exclusive remedy.* That is, if you have been injured on the job, in an accident which arose out of the course of your employment, then your lawsuit can only be filed within the workers' compensation laws of your state. However, if on-the-job sexual harassment is the cause of your injury(ies), then you may or may not be able to file your lawsuit within the workers' compensation legal system. In the state of New Mexico, sexual harassment survivors' injuries are not considered to have arisen as part of the employment process, so survivors are not considered injured workers, and must file their lawsuits within the body of law known as employment law. In other states, survivors can file in both systems.

I have seen sexual harassment survivors lose everything in their struggles with the tangle of these obscure, strange, and often incomprehensible systems. In California, I worked with a survivor who had attorneys for her workers' compensation case, attorneys from her union, attorneys for her employment law case, a claims examiner for the insurance carrier, a return-to-work coordinator for the employer, and me, the vocational rehabilitation counselor out of the workers' compensation system. I never did figure out who was on first, and I was not the one experiencing full-blown post-traumatic stress disorder symptoms of inability to trust, suspicion, hypervigilance, acute anxiety, lack of focus, inability to make a decision, and unrealistic expectations. This survivor lost her job, got a very poor workers' compensation lump sum settlement (barely enough to pay her debts), her vocational rehabilitation benefit, and her right to pursue her case in the employment law arena; all in the name of her lack of cooperation. She could never make a commitment to anything, because she was hooked on the idea that something better was just around the corner (e.g., The employer would give her job back and fire the perpetrator. The employer would get her a better job than she had before. She would get a $100,000 settlement).

Oh, and did I mention that if you don't use the workers' compensation law and the employment law options in the right order (when the moon is blue on alternative Tuesdays, or something), you may lose your rights in the other system?

The point is, *in order to survive in such a situation, you are going to have to make a decision to trust someone, something.* It may feel like taking a leap into total darkness, but if you do not make this decision, your power will be taken from you, and others will make decisions for you. If you have completed the work in this Workbook, your chances of choosing the right person or persons to trust are increased. You may still make the wrong decision, but if you have a vision for yourself, you will be able to go on with some of your dignity and integrity intact.

workers' compensation systems

Traumatic abuse survivors can find themselves inside workers' compensation systems in at least three ways. We have already discussed the first, sexual harassment. Some survivors may have experienced on-the-job traumas that are not sexual harassment, such as being held up at gunpoint while working as a grocery checker, being held hostage during a bank robbery, or seeing a co-worker die in an accident at work. These experiences, in and of themselves, can create post-traumatic stress disorder. Other survivors may have experienced the more common injuries such as cumulative trauma injuries to their wrists from continuous work at a computer keyboard, back injuries from too much heavy lifting, or knee injuries from a fall. Some physical injuries can also produce psychological trauma.

If you are a traumatic abuse survivor who has not done much healing prior to an industrial injury of any kind, you may find that your response to the industrial injury is overwhelming in its impact upon you physically and psychologically. All your past feelings of loss and betrayal may rise up like demons. You may be told that the objective or physical findings of the doctors are not consistent with the pain levels you are reporting. You may find yourself abusing prescription drugs and/or self-medicating for pain with illegal drugs or alcohol.

It is my experience that a physical injury of any sort, no matter how minor it may appear, has a profound effect upon us all. The integrity of our bodies has been violated. If we have not healed, or are not in a process of healing, from our traumatic abuse experience(s), then our ability to manage such a violation well is doubtful. If your industrial injury is another traumatic experience piled on top of your abuse history, you ability to manage will be shaky indeed. If this is your situation, then it will be your task to get on with the work of healing your trauma at the same time you are getting on with the work of healing your industrial injury.

Workers' compensation law refers to a principle of *preexisting conditions*. That is, employers (insurance carriers) are not obligated to provide benefits for conditions resulting from past injuries. This means that you are on your own in managing the healing from the traumatic abuse of your past, while going through the struggle to obtain the workers' compensation benefits and services owed to you. And, I promise, it will be a struggle. The job of employers and their agents, insurance carriers, is to provide the workers' compensation benefit to their injured workers in the most efficient manner, with the minimum amount of cost to them. This may or may not be in your best interest, but if you think your employer or the insurance carrier is acting in your best interests, then you are deluded. Perhaps they should act for your benefit, but should is a word for how we would like things to be, and not what is.

Workers' compensation benefits usually consist of payments for medical treatment, lawyer's fees, and perhaps vocational rehabilitation benefits and services. These benefits vary from state to state according to the laws of each state. In the late 80s, state governments launched an assault on the vocational rehabilitation benefit in the name of workers' compensation reform. Therefore, what the vocational rehabilitation benefit is in your state may be anybody's guess, since this so-called *reform* process is continuing into the 90s. The vocational rehabilitation benefit usually consists of some support for vocational testing, vocational counseling, training expenses — tuition, uniforms, books, supplies, and tools — resume development, and job search assistance. In Nevada, injured workers were entitled to 12 months of vocational rehabilitation maximum. In California, time in a vocational rehabilitation plan was negotiated in sometimes tedious and bitter quarrels, but the rule of thumb was one year or less. New Mexico no longer has a formal vocational rehabilitation benefit. All of this is changing as I write. Once again, I caution you to be very clear about your options before you make a decision as to the use of this benefit in your state, or the decision to fight to get it.

The value of your Management by Objective Career and Life Plan Statement and its companion, the Ten-year Plan, should be obvious here, because most workers' compensation systems are not going to provide you with all that you need. If there is a vocational rehabilitation benefit, you may want to drop it into your life weaving as an accent, a splash of color to represent that six months of computer training at the local business college. (The benefit did not allow you to get your bachelor's degree, but it did get you that good part-time job which allows you to go for your Ten-year Plan.) If you just got medical treatment, good. That gets woven into the pre-vocational portion of your career and life plan. If you got a lump sum settlement, then you can use your plan to figure out how best to use that money after settling the debts you probably now have.

TIP

Again, remember the *Take-the-money-and-run-principle*. The workers' compensation system will not save you no matter how much you think it should. I recommend adopting an attitude of gratitude in this situation, just because the prevention of psychic wear and tear is worth the trouble of doing so. A suggested affirmation is that whenever you get a workers' compensation check, tuition costs paid, physical therapy covered; you thank the universe as in: *I, (name) thank the abundance of the universe for giving me what I need today.*

employment law

Employment law covers a wide spectrum which includes laws on age, disability, racial, and gender discrimination. Sex discrimination and sexual harassment laws are included within this category of law. All of these laws build upon each other, and intersect in complex ways in legislative and case law. They are laws which allow civil suits to be filed in state and federal courts for lost wages, compensation for expenses incurred as the result of discrimination or injury, and in some situations, for noneconomic damages such as pain and suffering, loss of pleasure of life.

The determination of damages in these cases is quite similar to processes used in personal injury law cases. These are cases which involve automobile accidents and other disasters resulting in injury and/or death. Vocational experts are frequently used in personal injury cases in order to determine if the plaintiff has the ability to return to work or benefit from a vocational rehabilitation process; to create life care plans for those whose disabilities severely limit or destroy the ability to work at all; and to examine past and future earning capacity pre- and post-injury.

Vocational experts have rarely been used in sexual harassment and/or civil incest and civil sexual assault cases. Therefore, the vocational rehabilitation analysis, which is based on examining the relationships between work and disability for possible vocational impairment, has rarely been applied. In my opinion, this is because *a woman's status as a worker is still not recognized in our society, and because the injuries sustained by women as a result of traumatic abuse are still not considered serious injuries.*

Even in personal injury cases, an injured woman is less likely to have her past and future lost earning capacity examined, her potentiality for benefiting from vocational rehabilitation evaluated, and her status as a worker respected. She is more likely to be given damages for cosmetic disfigurement and psychological distress. The attitudes of judges, attorneys, and juries have apparently not caught up with the reality. Women work. They work at home, and they work in the waged work world in ever-increasing numbers.

Therefore, your Management by Objective Career and Life Plan and the Ten-year Plan will help you sustain your identity as a worker in a sexual harassment lawsuit where the struggle over the issues in the lawsuit will focus on your sexual identity rather than on your work identity. The work in this Workbook will help you sort out the sexual identity issues from the work identity issues. The sexual identity issues are so powerful, and the tendency in our society to deny women's status as workers is so ingrained, that you may find yourself and your own attorney swept away into confusion and doubt. Insist that an evaluation of the vocational impairment created by sexual harassment be done. This will change the focus, and get the spotlight onto the damage done to your worklife rather than some voyeuristic excursion into your sexual habits, tastes, and orientation.

Sexual harassment cases seem to have an infinite number of paths your attorney can take to file the lawsuit, methods of appealing decisions, and choices in which laws to use. The attorneys representing the employer also have these options.

Therefore, in dealing with sexual harassment and sex discrimination cases, it is probably wisest to adopt a back-at-the-loom attitude, or a get-on-with-the-business-of-weaving-your life approach. This is because such cases can drag on for months and years before reaching any sort of conclusion. Such cases can even extend beyond a Ten-year Plan (or feel that way). Therefore, don't put your life on hold. Get healing. Get moving.

civil incest and molestation lawsuits

In the 80s and early 90s, the media went into a feeding frenzy over the sensational civil molestation lawsuits brought by molestation survivors against Catholic priests. The time limitations for filing lawsuits against perpetrators of incest by adult survivors was extended in many states by the end of the 80s. A television movie was made about the California case where an adult survivor remembered not only being sexually abused by her father, but the murder of her childhood friend, a murder he committed in her presence. He was convicted of this crime, based on her retrieved memories.

Backlash against this assertion of rights by incest and molestation survivors has, not surprisingly, also emerged. The media has responded by giving these reactionary forces equal time in some sort of notion of journalistic integrity. Even Oprah Winfrey allowed the people from the False Memory Syndrome Foundation (FMSF) to shout and scream their lies and denials on national television. Facts seem to have no impact on these folks. For example on *Oprah!*, Ellen Bass, one of the coauthors of the classic book, *The Courage to Heal*, said repeatedly that the book does not advise anyone to sue their parents. The FMSF representative ignored her completely, and screamed the words, *"suing your parents"* in a tone of voice which suggested that such an action is the utmost in evil.

Ann Landers recently published a letter from the FMSF people with no rejoinder, no comments from her regarding their integrity, which would indicate that she respects their point of view.

The woman who founded FMSF is Pamela Freyd, the mother of Jennifer J. Freyd, a professor of psychology at the University of Oregon. Dr. Freyd has had to bear the pain and humiliation of her parents' claim, in the national media, that she has falsely accused her father of childhood sexual abuse. In August of 1993, Dr. Freyd broke her silence by presenting her paper, *Theoretical and Personal Perspectives on the Delayed Memory Debate,* at The Center for Mental Health at Foote Hospital's Continuing Education Conference: Controversies Around Recovered Memories of Incest and Ritualistic Abuse, in Ann Arbor, Michigan. Dr. Freyd sees FMSF as an organization which weaves together many strands. "One strand is my parents' need to deny my memories, a need so strong that they founded FSMF so shortly after I went into therapy. Denial of child sexual abuse is as old as child sexual abuse.... . There are many other strands that enter this knot. I believe one strand could be called the backlash to a new human rights movement — the children's rights movement."

If you are an incest or molestation survivor considering filing a civil
suit, you will find yourself dealing
with the chaos and confusion this organization has caused. Attorneys are
taking this all very seriously even
though there is no such diagnosis as
"false memory syndrome" in any recognized psychiatric or psychological

> **TIP**
> Dr. Freyd's paper can be ob-
> tained from The Making the Connec-
> tions Intercultural Network for $5.00.
> Make your check to The Union Insti-
> tute Center for Women and send it to
> 86 Monte Alto Road, Santa Fe, NM
> 87505.

literature such as the *Diagnostic & Statistical Manual of Mental Disorders* as published by the American Psychiatric Association.

The message of the FMSF is that therapists somehow "create" the memories of
sexual abuse reported to them by adult survivors. Dr. Freyd notes that, "Therapists
get blamed for memories of incest, in a way that reminds me of a tendency to shoot
the messenger." As a vocational expert, I would add that the FMSF assault on therapists is also an assault against an occupation dominated by women, an assault on
women's work. This assault escalates the discrediting of women's revelations regarding sexual assault to a new level. It is very similar to the attack on adult females
who report rape and/or sexual harassment on the job or in an educational setting.

The filing of a civil suit in incest, molestation, and rape cases will be fraught
with all the difficulties described in domestic tort and sexual harassment cases. Since
these cases are not brought forward as frequently as personal injury or divorce cases,
you will probably have a difficult time locating an attorney who is willing to take
such a case. Experts in post-traumatic stress disorder may not be easy to locate, and
the idea that incest or molestation can create disability leading to vocational impairment is still considered a radically new idea. What this means is that almost each
new case filed breaks new ground legally and socially.

RESOURCES – Crnich, J. E. & Crnich, K. A. (1992). *Shifting the Burden of Truth:
Suing Child Sexual Abusers–A Legal Guide for Survivors and Their Supporters.*
Lake Oswego, Oregon: Recollex Publishing. *Legal Resource Kit: Incest and Child
Sexual Abuse*, NOW Legal Defense and Education Fund, 99 Hudson Street, New
York, NY 10013-2815, (212) 925-6635 FAX (212) 226-1066.

I neither encourage you to, nor discourage you from, filing such lawsuits. However, you have a right to be informed about all your options. You have a right to
decide if you want to be a pioneer, a leader in the new human rights movement —
the children's rights movement.

Backlash is always a sign of success. That is, if the credibility of traumatic abuse
survivors had not reached new levels in the past three decades in the fields of law,
psychiatry, and psychology, we would not see this overwrought reaction. We would
simply be ignored. Perhaps the most important lesson of backlash is to understand
that it cannot be fought by individuals. Only the bonding together of survivors has
created a children's rights movement, a rape crisis movement, a battered women's
movement, and only our continued efforts together will defeat this latest version of

backlash. In fact, the attack of FMSF should be seen as an attack on these movements, and not on you as an individual survivor.

Any attack on your right to exercise *your legal right to sue* (even your parents), should be viewed as an assault against your fundamental civil liberties and your rights as a human being to a life free from abuse. Your Management by Objective Career and Life Plan and your Ten-year Plan are statements that your life has meaning and significance, that you have a right to weave your life into the pattern best for you. No one, not even your parents, has the right to *your* life. Abuse takes away our sense of ourselves as unique and irreplaceable beings. Our journey back to this birthright is sacred.

> **TIP**
> A suggested affirmation in the decision making process in this situation is, I, (name), am the weaver of my own life pattern.

civil sexual assault lawsuits

The statistically vulnerable years for rape are between the ages of 13 and 26 years (Russell, 1984). Unfortunately, the statue of limitations for the filing of a civil suit in a rape case may be exceeded by the time you have decided that such a lawsuit is appropriate. The years between the ages of 13 and 26 years are also prime years for vocational exploration, discovery, and decision-making. These are the years we enter junior high and high school, go to college or trade school, or enter the waged labor market for our first full-time jobs. Sexual assault during these years can have long-lasting and devastating effects on our vocational development. Results reported to me by clients include dropping out of school, giving up artistic pursuits such as singing, painting, writing; and marrying suddenly (sometimes inappropriately). Since most rape survivors do not connect their vocational decision-making to their experience of rape, they will then blame and criticize themselves for not fulfilling their vocational and creative goals.

Little research has been conducted on the effects of acquaintance rape on the work lives of young women enrolled in college at the time of the rape. My preliminary discussions with the staff of women's centers on college campuses reveals that it is not unusual for these young women to drop out of school and never return. There is no provision for helping a woman to manage her financial aid arrangements while trying to handle her rape trauma. This can mean that not only does she have to drop out of school, but she may not be able to return because there is no money to help her with her educational expenses. College administrations have no method of assisting a woman who is facing her alleged rapist in the classroom, or the dormitory, transfer to another class, dormitory, or even college campus. The assistance extended is largely counseling and services from the student health center. Although these are vital and basic services, the damage to the vocational potential and vocational aspirations of the rape survivor are not addressed even though the purpose of her presence on a college campus is the realization of her potential and aspirations.

Whether your rape experience has been recent or years ago, chances are that it has had an impact on your dreams for your life. You may wish to contact your local rape crisis center to get the name of an attorney who can advise you as to your rights in filing a civil suit for damages to your vocational aspirations and potential. Whether or not you have the right to sue, the exercises in this Workbook will allow you to untangle the threads and re-weave your life.

the Americans with Disabilities Act of 1990

This law was based on the Civil Rights Act of 1964 and the Rehabilitation Act of 1973. It is not an affirmative action law, but a civil rights law which has the potential to completely transform the workplace as we know it today. The Americans with Disabilities Act (ADA) is so new that there are still very few cases which have come down through the court system. This means that the interpretation of the law is not encrusted by years, decades, maybe centuries of case law decisions. In other words, now is the time to participate in the process of giving the ADA meaning.

What I mean by this is that laws are not just about the business of filing lawsuits and giving money to attorneys; laws are also statements about our society and what we expect from the members within it. In some ways, our awareness of laws and our subsequent actions which arise from this awareness are more important than any lawsuit. Lawsuits are for the purpose of forcing people to do things, or pay up for damages, or for punishment of wrongdoers. Acting as if the law is how we are to behave is a more positive, proactive approach.

The ADA offers both an opportunity and a challenge to traumatic abuse survivors. The opportunity is to take the law at its word when it defines mental and emotional disorders as disabilities which can impair our ability to function in the waged work world. That is, post-traumatic stress disorder symptoms can create vocational barriers and impairments which might need accommodation in the new workplace. A reasonable accommodation might be as simple as providing extra time for learning the job for those trauma survivors whose ability to concentrate has been damaged. The need for flex time or time off the job (to be made up at another time) to attend therapy sessions for the management of post-traumatic stress disorder is another example. The opportunity lies in the creativity of trauma survivors in assessing what they need in the workplace to make working possible for themselves.

The challenge lies in communicating both the need for the accommodation and the nature of the accommodation to the employer. Trauma survivors may be understandably be reluctant, or unable, to explain their disability to the employer. However, the ADA requires that the person with the disability request the reasonable accommodation.

If you have completed the exercises in this Workbook, you are in the forefront of the implementation of this new law because you have named your trauma, discovered the vocational impairment your trauma has created for you, and made a plan to heal both your trauma and your vocational impairment. Your ability to request a reasonable accommodation from an employer is probably greater than any expert now on the scene.

Your accomplishment is heroic. If the promise of the ADA to dispel stereotypes and assumptions about disabilities, and to ensure equality of opportunity, full participation, independent living, and economic self-sufficiency is ever to become reality, it is women like you who will lead the way.

RESOURCE – *The Edge of A Large Hole: Writings on the Request for Reasonable Accommodation Under the Americans with Disabilities Act of 1990* by Patricia A. Murphy. Center for Research on Women and Gender, UIC, 1640 W. Roosevelt Road, Room 207 (M/C 980), Chicago, IL 60608, (312) 413-1924.

noneconomic damages awards or how our lives are about more than our earning capacities

> *The strategic inference should be clear: we must give voice to the hurting self, even when that hurting self sounds like a child rather than an adult; even when the hurting self voices "trivial" complaints; even when the hurting self is ambivalent toward the harm; and even when (especially when) the hurting self is talking a language not heard in public discourse. Only by so doing will we ourselves become aware of the meaning of the suffering in our lives, and its contingency in our history. Only when we understand the contingency of that pain will we be free to address it and through legal tools to change the conditions that cause it.*
>
> Robin West, 1993, p. 184

Noneconomic damage awards refer to awards given for emotional distress, pain and suffering, and/or loss of pleasure in life. The Civil Rights Act of 1991 states that compensatory damages may be awarded for future pecuniary losses, emotional pain, suffering, inconvenience, mental anguish, loss of enjoyment of life, and other nonpecuniary losses. This Act means that persons filing lawsuits in employment arenas such as sex discrimination, sex harassment, and Americans with Disabilities Act cases can now file for noneconomic damage awards. Such awards can also be awarded in domestic tort, civil sexual assault, civil incest, and personal injury cases. If a lawsuit is filed in state courts, the laws of each state will determine the limits and definitions for such damages.

If the idea that traumatic abuse can create disability leading to damaged earning capacities for survivors is startling, then the idea that women have the right to damage awards based on the loss of the enjoyment of their lives (including their work lives) is equivalent to a mental earthquake. Acceptance of this idea means that traumatic abuse survivors cannot be reduced to the status of victims. It means that a woman's whole life must be honored, her right to pleasure in her life, to dignity, to a quality life.

Since these ideas are so unknown in most courts of law, an expert will probably be called upon to develop arguments to support the demand for damages. These experts may include psychologists to testify to emotional distress, vocational experts to testify to the hedonic or noneconomic damage caused by the loss of occupations, economists to testify to the actual amount of such awards. The economist will make her calculations based on the work of the other experts (psychologists and/or vocational experts).

With the exception of 1988 report *Estimating the Cost of Sexual Harassment to the Fortune 500 Service and Manufacturing Firms* (Klein, 1988), there are little data available on the costs of the traumatic abuse of women to the society at large. Such data are now being sought and it is my expectation that within the next decade we will have more information to use in formulating how noneconomic damage awards should be developed in traumatic abuse lawsuits. The Klein report estimates that the cost of turnover of non-managerial employees is 1/4th of their average annual wage, including benefits.

In a recent sex harassment case, I used the Klein report and drew upon other authorities (Berla, Brookshire, & Smith, 1990 for a general conceptual approach and Magrowski, 1991, for thoughts on the loss of occupations) to justify a noneconomic damage award to a sex harassment survivor in the amount of *$122,354 above and beyond the damage to her future* earning capacity which was calculated at a range between $199,857 to $236,631.

Nothing — no amount of money — can ever make up for the anguish and humiliation of traumatic abuse. Perhaps the most important aspect of this kind of damage award is the acknowledgment it brings to the "hurting self." Without this acknowledgment, how will we ever bring about change not only for ourselves, but for every person?

Therefore if you have decided to file a lawsuit, remember that you have a right to explore the possibility of receiving a noneconomic damage award. You have the right to have your "hurting self" acknowledged.

It is fitting that the Workbook should conclude with this issue because, noneconomic damages awards perhaps speak to the underlying theme of all of the work you have completed here. That is, your life, *in and of itself*, is unique, precious, and valuable.

From one weaver to another—blessings.

Patricia A. Murphy

references and
suggested readings

Allen, P. G. (1986). *The sacred hoop: Recovering the feminine in American Indian traditions.* Boston: Beacon Press.

Allen, P. G. (Ed.) (1989). *Spider women's granddaughters: Traditional tales and contemporary writing by native American women.* New York: Fawcett Columbine.

Allison, M. (1993, March/April). Exploring the link between violence and brain injury.*Headline.*

American Medical Association. (1992, March). *Diagnostic and treatment guidelines on domestic violence.* Chicago: Author.

American Psychiatric Association. (1987). *Diagnostic and statistical manual of mental disorders* (3rd ed., rev.). Washington, DC: Author.

Anzaldua, G. (Ed.). 1990. *Making face, making soul: Haciendo caras.* San Francisco: Aunt Lute Foundation Books.

Barry, K. (1979). *Female sexual slavery.* New York: New York University Press.

Barry, K. (1984). The network defines its issues: Theory, evidence, and analysis of female sexual slavery. In K. Barry, C. Bunch, & S. Casteley (Eds.). *International feminism: Networking against female sexual slavery* (pp. 32-48). New York: The International Women's Tribune Centre, Inc.

Bart, P. B., & Moran, E. G. (Eds.) (1993). *Violence against women: The bloody footprints.* Newbury Park, CA: Sage Publications.

Bartlett, K. T. (1991). Feminist legal methods. In K. T. Bartlett & R. Kennedy (Eds.),*New perspectives on law, culture, and society* (p. 393). Boulder, CO: Westview Press, Inc.

Bass, E., & Davis, L. (1988). *The courage to heal: A guide for women survivors of child sexual abuse.* New York: Perennial Library.

Bass, E., & Davis, L. (1994). *The courage to heal: A guide for women survivors of child sexual abuse,* third edition. New York: Perennial Library.

Belenky, M. F., Clinchy, B. M., Goldberger, N. R., & Tarule, J. M. (1986). *Women's ways of knowing: The development of self, voice, and mind.* New York: Basic Books.

Berla, E. P., Brookshire, M. L., & Smith, S. V. (1990). Hedonic damages and personal injury: A conceptual approach. *Journal of Forensic Economics.*3(1), 1-8.

Bolles, R. N. (1992). *The 1992 what color is your parachute?* Berkeley, CA: Ten Speed Press.

Bower, B. (1991, August 31). Women's trail of tears, (p. 141).*Science News.*

Brown, L. S. (1992). A feminist critique of the personality disorders. In L. A. Brown, L. A. & M. Ballou (Eds.), *Personality and psychopathology: Feminist reappraisals*(pp. 206-228). New York: The Guilford Press.

Brown, W. (1992, Spring). Finding the man in the state.*Feminist Studies,* 18(1): 7-34.

Burgess, A. W., & Holmstrom, L. L. (1979). *Rape: Crisis and recovery.* Bowie, Maryland: Brady Co.

Burgess, A. W., & Holmstrom, L. L. (1985). Rape trauma syndrome and post traumatic stress response. In A. W. Burgess, (Ed.). *Rape and sexual assault: A research handbook*(pp. 46-60). New York: Garland Publishing, Inc.

Campbell, J. (1990, December). Battered woman syndrome: A critical review. *Violence Update,* pp. 1, 4, 10-11.

Caputi, J. (1987). *The age of sex crime.* Bowling Green, OH: Bowling Green State University Press.

Caputi, J. (1993). *Gossips, gorgons, and crones: The fates of the earth.* Santa Fe, NM: Bear & Company.

Chang, J. (1991). *Wild swans: Three daughters of China.* New York: Anchor Books.

Chicago, J. (1977). *Through the flower: My struggle as a woman artist.* Garden City, New York: Anchor Books.

Chicago, J. (1979). *The dinner party: A symbol of our heritage.* Garden City, New York: Anchor Books.

Chicago, J. (1980). *Embroidering our heritage: The dinner party needlework.* Garden City, New York: Anchor Books.

Chicago, J. (1985). *The birth project.* Garden City, New York: Doubleday & Company.

Chicago, J. (1993). *The holocaust project: From darkness into light.* Garden City, NY: Anchor Books.

Collier, R. J. (1993, April 26). The stigma of mental illness, (p. 16). *Newsweek.*

Collins, P. H. (1990). *Black feminist thought: Knowledge, consciousness, and the politics of empowerment.* New York: Routledge.

Copper, B. (1988). *Over the hill: Reflections on ageism between women.* Freedom, CA: The Crossing Press.

Crnich, J. E., & Crnich, K. A. (1992). *Shifting the burden of truth: Suing child sexual abusers–a legal guide for survivors and their supporters.* Lake Oswego, OR: Recollex Publishing.

Crow Dog, M., & Erdoes, R. (1990). *Lakota Woman.* New York: Harper Perennial.

Dan, A. J., & Hemphill, S. T. (1993). Women's health. *The 1993 Medical and Health Annual.* Chicago: Encyclopedia Britannica, Inc.

Dan, A. J. (Ed.) (1994). *Reframing women's health: Multidisciplinary research and practice.* Thousand Oaks, CA: Sage Publications, Inc.

Dan, A. J. (Ed.) (1994, July 20-29). *Report of framing women's health: An intensive summer institute.* Chicago: UIC Center for Research on Women and Gender.

Davis, L. (1990). *The courage to heal workbook for women and men survivors of child sexual abuse.* New York: Perennial Library.

Deutsch, P., & Sawyer, H. W. (1992). *A guide to rehabilitation.* New York: Ahab Press, Inc.

Enloe, C. (1989). *Making feminist sense of international politics: Bananas, beach & bases.* Berkeley, CA: University of California Press.

Evans, L. J. (1978). Sexual harassment: Women's hidden occupational hazard. In J. R. Chapman & M. Gates (Eds.), *The victimization of women* (pp. 203-223). Newbury Park, CA: Sage Publications.

Evans, P. (1992). *The verbally abusive relationship: How to recognize it and how to respond.* Holbrook, MA: Bob Adams, Inc.

Field, T. F. (Ed.). (1989). The value and worth of housewives and household activities. *The Professional Reader, 1,* 1. Athens, GA: Elliott & Fitzpatrick.

Finkelhor, D., & Yllo, K. (1985). *License to rape: Sexual abuse of wives.* New York: Holt, Rinehart and Winston.

Fitzgerald, L. G., & Crites, J. O. (1980). Toward a career psychology of women: What do we know? What do we need to know? *Journal of Counseling Psychology, Vol. 27,* no. 1, p. 44.

Fogel, R. W. (1989). *Without consent or contract: The rise and fall of American slavery.* New York: W. W. Norton.

Fuentes, A., & Ehrenreich, B. (1983). *Women in the global factory.* Boston: South End Press.

Gilligan, C., Lyons, N. P., & Hanmer, T. J. (Eds.) (1990). *Making connections: The relational worlds of adolescent girls at Emma Willard School.* Cambridge, MA: Harvard University Press.

Goldberg, N. (1990). *Wild mind: Living the writer's life.* New York: Bantam Books.

Goldberg, N. (1993). *Long quiet highway: Waking up in America.* New York: Bantam Books.

Grothaus, R. S. (1985). Abuse of women with disabilities. In S. E. Browne, D. Connors, & N. Stern (Eds.), *With the power of each breath: A disabled women's anthology.* (pp. 124-130). Pittsburgh: Cleis Press.

Gutek, B. A., & Larwood, L. (Eds.) (1989). *Women's career development.* Newbury Park, CA: Sage Publications.

Hanna, W. J., & Rogovsky, E. (1992, Winter). On the situation of African-American women with physical disabilities. *Journal of Applied Rehabilitation Counseling,* (23)4: 39-45.

Hay, L. L. (1988). *Heal your body: The mental causes for physical illness and the metaphysical way to overcome them.* Santa Monica, CA: Hay House, Inc.

Heilbrun, C. G. (1988). *Writing a woman's life.* New York: W. W. Norton & Company.

Herman, J. L. (1992). *Trauma and Recovery: The aftermath of violence — from domestic abuse to political terror.* New York: Basic Books.

Higgins, P. C. (1992). *Making disability: Exploring the social transformation of human variation.* Springfield, IL: Charles C. Thomas Publisher.

Hines, D. C. (1989, Summer). Rape and the inner lives of Black women in the Middle West: Preliminary thoughts on the culture of dissemblance. *Signs: Journal of Women in Culture and Society,* 14(4): 912-920.

Hooks, B. (1989, July/August). Reflections on Race and Sex. *Z Magazine, Vol 1,* no. 1-8, P. 57.

Hyer, S. (1993). *Women's work: The art of Pablita Velarde.* Santa Fe, NM: The Wheelwright Museum of the American Indian.

Hyman, B. (1993, April). *The economic consequences of child sexual abuse in women.* Washington, DC: National Clearinghouse on Child Abuse & Neglect.

Johnson T. L. (1993). A women's health research agenda.*Journal of Women's Health,* (2)-2: 95-98.

Jones, S. (1993). *Counselor's survey of employment characteristics of women using Illinois battered women shelters.* (Unpublished survey results.) Wheaton, IL: Wheaton Extension Center.

Karp, L., & Karp, C. L. (1989). *Domestic torts: Family violence, conflict and sexual abuse.* Colorado Springs, CO: Shepard's/McGraw-Hill, Inc.

Karp, L. & Karp, C. L. (1993, June). *Domestic torts: Family violence, conflict and sexual abuse. Cumulative Supplement.* Colorado Spring, CO: Shepard's/McGraw-Hill, Inc.

Klein, F. (1988, November). *The 1988 Working Woman sexual harassment survey: Executive report.* Cambridge: Author.

Koss, M. P. (1992, September). Medical consequences of rape. *Violence Update,* pp. 1, 9-11).

Koss, M. P., & Heslet, L. (1992, September). Somatic consequences of violence against women. *Archives of Family Medicine. Vol 1,* p. 53.

Kurz, D., & Stark, E. (1988). Not-so-benign neglect: The medical response to battering. In K. Yllo & M. Bograd, (Eds.), *Feminist perspectives on wife abuse* (pp. 249-265). Newbury Park, CA: Sage Publications.

Lippard, L. R. (1990). Uninvited guests: How Washington lost "The Dinner Party." *Art in America,* 39-49.

Lloyd, S. (1994, January). *The effects of violence on work and family.* Evanston, IL: Center for Urban Affairs and Policy Research, Northwestern University.

Lorde, A. (1984). *Sister outsider.* Freedom, CA: The Crossing Press.

MacKinnon, C. A. (1987). *Feminism unmodified: Discourses on life and law.* Cambridge, MA: Harvard University Press.

Magrowski, J. F. (1991, March). Future vocational expert testimony on hedonics (pp. 72-28)*Monograph #1: The vocational expert's testimony.* Skokie, IL: American Board of Vocational Experts.

Mancusco, L. L (1993, June). *Reasonable accommodations for workers with psychiatric disabilities.* Sacramento, CA: California Department of Mental Health.

Martz, S. (Ed.). (1990). *If I had a hammer: Women's work in poetry, fiction, and photographs.* Watsonville, CA: Papier-Mache Press.

McFarlane, J., Parker, B., Soeken, K., & Bullock, L. (1992, June 17). Assessing for abuse during pregnancy: Severity and frequency of injuries and associated entry into prenatal care.*Journal of the American Medical Association, Vol. 267,* No. 23, 3176-3178.

McConnell, J. E. (1992, Spring). Beyond metaphor: Battered women, involuntary servitude, and the thirteenth amendment. *Yale Journal of Law and Feminism, 4(2),* 207-253.

McNeil, J. (1983). *Labor force status and other characteristics of persons with a work disability.* Washington, DC: U. S. Department of Commerce, Bureau of the Census.

Miller, A. (1990). *Banished knowledge: Facing childhood injuries.* New York: Anchor Books.

Morales, A. L., & Morales, R. (1986). *Getting home alive.* Ithaca, NY: Firebrand Books.

Morgan, L. A. (1991). *After marriage ends: Economic consequences for midlife women.* Newbury Park, CA: Sage Publications, Inc.

Murphy, P. A. (1992, December 18). *Evaluation of lost earning capacity and vocational potential for Colleen S. Gibbins.* Santa Fe, NM: The Making the Connections Project.

Murphy, P. A. (1992). Taking an abuse history in the initial evaluation.*NARRPS Journal & News*, (7)-5: 187-191.

Murphy, P. A. (1993). *Making the connections: Women, work & abuse.* Delray Beach, FL: St. Lucie Press, Inc.

Murphy, P. A. (1994). *The edge of a large hole: Writings on the request for reasonable accommodation under the Americans with Disabilities Act of 1990.* Chicago: University of Illinois at Chicago Center for Research on Women and Gender.

National Clearinghouse for the Defence of Battered Women. (1993, December).*Know of any battered women who have been denied insurance benefits?* Double-time. Philadelphia: Author.

Neland, V. (undated). *CPA Handbook.* Portland OR: Council for Prostitution Alternatives.

Parrish, J. (1991). Reasonable accommodations for people with psychiatric disabilities.*Community Support Network News*, (p. 8). Boston: Center for Psychiatric Rehabilitation.

Parsons, E. R. (1985). Ethnicity and traumatic stress: The intersecting point in psychotherapy. In C. R. Figley (Ed.), *Trauma and its wake: The study and treatment of post-traumatic stress disorder* (pp. 314-335). New York: Brunner-Mazel.

Perera, S. B. (1981). *Descent to the goddess: A way of initiation for women.* Toronto: Inner City Books.

Rayman, P., & Allshouse, K. (1990, December). *Resiliency amidst inequity: Older women workers in an aging United States.* Southport, CT: Southport Institute for Policy Analysis.

Rich, A. (1979). *On lies, secrets, and silence: Selected prose 1966-1978.* New York: W. W. Norton.

Richardson, M. S. (1993). Work in people's lives: A location for counseling psychologists*Journal of Counseling Psychology*, (40)-4: 425-433.

Richie, B. E. (1994). Gender entrapment: An exploratory study. In A. J. Dan (Ed.)*Reframing women's health: Multidisciplinary research and practice.* (pp. 219-232). Thousand Oaks, CA: Sage Publications, Inc.

Root, M. P. P. (1992). Reconstructing the impact of trauma on personality. In L. A. Brown & M. Ballou (Eds.), *Personality and psychopathology: Feminist reappraisals* (pp. 229-266). New York: The Guilford Press.

Russell, D. E. H. (1984). *Sexual exploitation: Rape, child sexual abuse, and workplace harassment.* Thousand Oaks: Sage Publication.

Russell, D. E. H. (1990). *Rape in marriage.* Bloomington, IN: Indiana University Press.

Saxton, M. (1985). A peer counseling training program for disabled women: A tool for social and individual change. In M. J. Deegan & N. A. Brooks (Eds.), pp. 95-105.*Women and disability: The double handicap.* New Brunswick, NJ: Transaction, Inc.

Scalise, J. J. (Ed.). (1989, Fall). *The Professional Reader: Estimating Future Lost Earnings As a Consequence of Injury, 1(3).* Athens, GA: Elliot & Fitzpatrick.

Schechter, S. (1982). *Women and male violence: The visions and struggles of the battered women's movement.* Boston: South End Press.

Schmidt, J. J. Crimando, W., & Riggar, T. F. (1990).*Sexual harassment in the workplace: A trainer's guide.* Athens, GA: Elliott & Fitzpatrick.

Schriner, K. F. (1990, Spring). Why study disability policy?*Journal of Disability Policy Studies*, 1(1): 2-7.

Shapiro, J. P. (1993). *No pity: People with disabilities forging a new civil rights movement.* New York: Times Books.

Siegel, D. L. (1992). *Sexual harassment research and resources.* New York: The National Council for Research on Women.

Silko, L. M. (1978). *Ceremony.* New York: Signet.

Sjoo, M., & Mor, B. (1987). *The great cosmic mother: Rediscovering the religion of the earth.* San Francisco: Harper & Row.

Smolowe, J. (1992, June 29). What the doctor should do. *Time Magazine*, p. 57.

Spalter-Roth, R. M., Hartmann, H. I., & Andrews, L. (1992). *Combining work and welfare: An alternative antipoverty strategy.* Washington, DC: Institute for Women's Policy Research.

Spretnak, C. (1978). *Lost goddess of early Greece: A collection of pre-Hellenic mythology.* Berkeley, CA: Moon Books.

Social Security Administration. (1990, February). Vocational expert handbook. Sacramento, CA: Office of Hearings and Appeals.

Stone, M. (1979). *Ancient mirrors of womanhood: A treasury of goddess and heroine lore from around the world.* Boston: Beacon Press.

Strauss, M. A. , Gelles, R. J., & Steinmetz, S. K. (1981). *Behind closed doors: Violence in the American family.* Newbury Park, CA: Sage Publications.

Suarez de Balcazar, Y., Bradford, B., & Fawcett, S. B. (1988, Fall). Common concerns of disabled Americans: Issues and options, (pp. 29-35). *Social Policy.*

Through the Flower. (undated). *Information about Judy Chicago's The Dinner Party.* Santa Fe, NM: Author.

Trimble, M. R. (1985). Post-traumatic stress disorder: History of a concept. In C. R. Figley (Ed.), *Trauma and its wake: The study and treatment of post-traumatic stress disorder* (pp. 5-15). New York: Brunner-Mazel.

Tripp, L. (1994, November). President signs Violence Against Women Act. *National Now Times*, p. 2.

Tsushima, M. (1992, December 14). The Americans with Disabilities Act and the battered woman. *A Working Paper of the Making the Connections Project.* Santa Fe, NM: The Making the Connections Intercultural Network.

United States Congress, Office of Technology Assessment. (1994, March). *Psychiatric disabilities, employment, and the Americans with Disabilities Act.* Washington, DC: U.S. Government Printing Office.

United States Department of Commerce, Bureau of the Census. (1987, August). Male-Female Differences in Work Experience, Occupation, and Earnings: 1984. *Household economic studies, Series P-70, No. 10.* Washington, D.C.: Government Printing Office.

United States Department of Labor, Bureau of Labor Statistics. (1992-1993). *Occupational outlook handbook.* Indianapolis, IN: JIST Works, Inc.

United States Department of Labor, Bureau of Labor Statistics. (1986, February). *Worklife estimates: Effects of race and education. Bulletin 2254.* Author.

Valenzuela, L. (1991). Writing with the body. In J. Sternburg (Ed.), *The writer on her work, Volume II* (pp. 192-200). New York: W. W. Norton & Company.

Walker, A. (1980). One child of one's own: A meaningful digression with the work(s). In J. Sternburg (Ed.), *The writer on her work: Contemporary women writers reflect on their art and situation* (pp. 121-140). New York: W. W. Norton & Company.

Walker, A. (1992). *Possessing the secret of joy.* New York: Pocket Star Books.

Walker, L. E. (1979). *The battered woman.* New York: Harper & Row.

Walker, L. E. (1989). *Terrifying love: Why battered women kill and how society responds.* New York: Harper & Row

Waring, M. (1988). *If women counted: A new feminist economics.* San Francisco: Harper & Row.

Warshaw, C. (1993). Limitations of the medical model in the care of battered women. In P. B. Bart & E. G. Moran (Eds.), *Violence against women: The bloody footprints* (pp. 134-146). Newbury Park, CA: Sage Publications.

Warshaw, R. (1988). *I never called it rape: The MS. report on recognizing, fighting and surviving date and acquaintance rape.* New York: Harper & Row.

Watson, C. G., Juba, M. P., Manifold, V., Kucala, T., & Anderson, P. E. D. (1991, March). The PTSD interview: Rationale, description, reliability, and concurrent validity of a DSM-III based technique. *Journal of Clinical Psychology,* 47(2), 188.

Waxman, B. F. (1991). Hatred: The unacknowledged dimension in violence against disabled people. *Sexuality and Disability*, (9)-3: 185-197.

Wendell, S. (1989, Summer). Toward a feminist theory of disability. *Hypatia*, 4(2): 104-124.

West. R. (1993). *Narrative, authority and law.* Ann Arbor: University of Michigan Press.

Williams, G. J., & Money, J. (Eds.) (1980). *Traumatic abuse and neglect of children at home.* Baltimore: Johns Hopkins University Press.

Williams, P. J. (1991). *The alchemy of race and rights: Diary of a law professor.* Cambridge: Harvard University Press.

Zuckerman, D., Debehhan, K, & Moore, K. (1993). *The ADA and people with mental illness: A resource manual for employers.* Alexandria, VA: American Bar Association and National Mental Health Association.